WS 430

3683
1R.

HIP SCREENING IN TH
A PRACTICAL

To Caroline
and to
Rose, Hawys and Rhonwen

HIP SCREENING IN THE NEWBORN: A PRACTICAL GUIDE

(A practical guide for general practitioners, clinical medical officers, paediatric and orthopaedic trainees, health visitors, midwives, and other health professionals concerned with child health)

DAVID ANTHONY JONES

BSc(Hons), MCh(Wales), FRCS(Eng)

Consultant Paediatric Orthopaedic Surgeon,
Morriston Hospital, Swansea
Honorary Clinical Teacher in Orthopaedics,
University of Wales College of Medicine

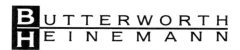

OXFORD   BOSTON   JOHANNESBURG   MELBOURNE   NEW DELHI   SINGAPORE

Butterworth-Heinemann
Linacre House, Jordan Hill, Oxford OX2 8DP
225 Wildwood Avenue, Woburn, MA 01801-2041
A division of Reed Educational and Professional Publishing Ltd

℞ A member of the Reed Elsevier plc group

First published 1998

British Library Cataloguing in Publication Data
A catalogue record for this book is available from the British Library

Library of Congress Cataloguing in Publication Data
A catalogue record for this book is available from the Library of Congress

ISBN 0 7506 2764 6

Printed and bound in Great Britain by MPG Books Ltd, Bodmin, Cornwall

CONTENTS

PREFACE

Congenital dislocation of the hip (CDH) remains as much of a problem today as it was when Ortolani and Barlow described tests which were widely acclaimed as the method by which this disease would be eradicated.

The problems are not quite the same, however, since the cases which now present late are never, or at least rarely, very late but the detection of cases between 3 and 6 months has led to difficult management decisions which we are only learning to cope with in a logical way.

The very term 'congenital dislocation of the hip' is no longer considered to be accurate for this disorder (or perhaps group of disorders). Some considerable time ago, both Somerville and (in a separate book) Wilkinson used the term 'congenital displacement of the hip'. Now the term 'developmental dysplasia of the hip' (DDH) is used because it recognises that the problem is not always a dislocation and also that it may develop and progress during the early months of life.

Regardless of what we call it, it can be defined as a congenitally determined developmental deformation of the hip joint in which the head of the femur is or may be partially or completely displaced from the acetabulum. In this book the methods of screening are described in a practical way on the 'cookbook' principle. Only one method of ultrasound screening will be described, because while the place of ultrasound in the management of early DDH is accepted, there is still great debate about its place in screening and it would be fair to say that it remains to be defined. The main purpose of this book is to bring together all the facts that the 'screener' and all those health professionals in the screening team need to have at their fingertips on a day to day basis in the clinical environment. At the same time it is hoped that it will provide much of the background information required for a deeper understanding of the principles involved. At regular intervals tips will be given and these will be highlighted in such a way that they are obvious to the reader and it is hoped that they will be of significant practical assistance.

David Anthony Jones

FOREWORD

by **Professor Brian McKibbin**
Emeritus Professor of Orthopaedic and Traumatic Surgery,
University of Wales, College of Medicine

Advances in medical treatment can arise in various ways. Sometimes these are dependent on entirely new discoveries, but often they are due to the perceptive combination of knowledge that has been long in existence. Screening for what is still widely known as congenital dislocation of the hip is a good example of this latter.

It has long been understood that the difficulty of treating this condition increases the longer reduction is delayed, due to the development of secondary anatomical changes. It has also been known for years that the diagnosis can usually be made soon after birth by simple clinical examination. The need for early treatment therefore seems obvious. Yet, it was not until the 1950s that Palmen and van Rosen extended this to the newborn period and introduced routine screening followed by simple splintage when a dislocation was identified.

The idea was rapidly adopted worldwide. In the heady days soon after the introduction of screening, it seemed as if the condition could be eliminated almost completely, like the earlier orthopaedic scourges of poliomyelitis and tuberculosis. Unfortunately, as in many other screening programmes, further experience began to cast doubt on this simple idea. Many unstable hips were identified and treated, often far more than the expected incidence of about 1 or 2 per 1000 births. Obviously, many normal children were being unnecessarily treated, but this was held to be a price worth paying for the sake of the genuine cases.

Unfortunately, even in the treated children, simple splintage did not always suffice, and a proportion continued to need surgical treatment. In addition, in some studies, the incidence of late presentation in the rest of the population stubbornly refused to fall. This prompted the uncomfortable conclusion that the children who were being identified and treated early were suffering only from physiological laxity of the joint capsule that would correct itself. The genuine cases were either being missed or, even if detected, were failing to respond to simple splintage. In many series, when the number of missed cases was added to those requiring surgery, the resulting figure came to something very close to the natural incidence of the condition.

This led some surgeons to conclude that in the 'genuine' cases there were anatomical abnormalities that would frustrate simple splintage. It was even suggested that although the children should be screened, no treatment should be given until 12 months later. By this time the physiological cases would have recovered while the 'genuine' could be treated by a simple operation at that still comparatively early stage. Others rejected these conclusions and argued that the original arguments remained sound and that the failures were due to inadequate skill in the application of the screening programme. However, few would argue that the problem is as simple as was originally thought. Hence the need for a book of this type, and the reader will be guided around the various pitfalls in the following pages.

However, although these conflicting views continue, nothing should be allowed to obscure the fact that the introduction of hip screening has proved to be a great good overall. Because of it, there is now general awareness of the importance of early treatment, so that even if a case is missed by a screening programme it is unlikely to continue unnoticed until there is a major surgical problem. Late cases, recognised only when a child has been limping for months and years, are now fortunately a rarity. Nevertheless, they have not been eliminated completely, and while they remain, efforts must continue to refine both the screening process and the subsequent treatment.

ACKNOWLEDGEMENTS

The library, and in particular Mrs Anne Powell, have been of enormous assistance to me in all the years of research on the subject of DDH, as well as in the preparation for this book. I would like to acknowledge the help of the postgraduate medical centre, and in particular Mrs Sandra Williams. In addition, the secretarial help of Mrs Janet Lodwig and Mrs Wendy Harris is acknowledged. My DDH clinics are held at the Philip's Parade Clinic under the supervision of Mrs Cynthia Elkes-Jones and her staff. Without their help I could not have gained the necessary information and experience to write about this subject. I have to thank generations of paediatric SHOs from Morriston and, more recently, Singleton Hospital for putting up with what they must at times have considered an over-enthusiastic approach! The consultant paediatricians have supported my efforts in every way and I thank them. My thanks are also due to Dr Niels Powell for setting up an ultrasound screening service for Swansea and Dr Tony Power for doing arthrograms on the late cases (the majority of which are from outside our geographical area).

1

Screening basics

Introduction

Screening involves a quite different relationship between the health professional and the patient than the normal clinical encounter to which we have become accustomed. The usual situation is that the patient or parents of the patient report a symptom or sign and they come to request further information or treatment. With screening, however, the health professional group is looking at a population which considers itself to be normal. The initiation of the process is by the profession and not the patient and it is based on the fact that there is a disease which the patient may be harbouring in an asymptomatic form and it is to the benefit of the patient for that disease process to be identified.

> **Tip**
>
> **Sometimes the word screening can be confused with the same word used in an X-ray context. Population screening (about which we are talking) has got nothing to do with X-ray screening.**

Screening is only one of the many methods of disease prevention, and is therefore popular with the general public and with politicians; both of these groups consider screening to be 'good'. Later in this book (see Chapter 7) the ethical considerations which should be applied to any screening programme will be considered in detail but at this stage it should simply be emphasised that it must be ascertained that the parents of the babies being screened for developmental dysplasia of the hip (DDH) really understand the process and therefore could be considered to have given informed consent. It is very rare for a parent to refuse screening procedures but it is also uncommon, on a national basis, for the parents to be given any detailed explanation of the process.

The parents themselves can be of great practical help in the screening

> **Tip**
>
> Take parental concern *very* seriously!
>   When we first started our studies in Swansea, one of the paediatric SHOs (Dr Rosser) diligently reviewed the notes of all past patients who had required inpatient treatment for DDH. One of my most lasting memories of observing these notes was the number of occasions when parents kept insisting there was an abnormality but they kept getting reassurance that all was well. For either of the parents to have been a member of the medical or nursing professions seemed to be a particular disadvantage in getting their concerns taken seriously!
>   It has altered my practice in that I now regard parental concern as a risk factor and at any sign of it in the neonatal period I will order a ultrasound scan or, if appropriate, an X-ray.

process and their concerns must be taken seriously. This applies especially in identifying babies who have special risk factors for DDH, e.g. breech position *in utero* or a family history, details which can sometimes be overlooked by a busy house doctor. A simple information leaflet (see Figure 7.1) given to all parents in the antenatal stage may be considered advisable at that stage, but this is essential at the time of screening.

> **Tip**
>
> Not only is it proper in terms of fully informed consent to tell parents that the clinical tests are not 100% reliable, it also gives you the reason and the opportunity to explain why it is important for tests to be repeated at a later date.

Conditions for any screening programme

When consideration is being given to setting up a screening programme for a disease it is very important to consider the generally accepted criteria which should be satisfied. They are related to the disease and the test.

Disease criteria

1. The disease must be significant.
2. The incidence must be reasonably high.
3. Treatment must be feasible.
4. Treatment must be available.

Test criteria

1. It must be reliable.
2. It must be acceptable.
3. Its cost must be reasonable.

Screening as a filtration system

For those not used to the concept of screening, it can be likened to a filtration system such as the one shown in Figure 1.1.

In some childhood diseases there is a specific test which can easily be done on the urine so that it is possible to tell on a single examination whether a child has the disease phenylketonuria, which is a metabolic

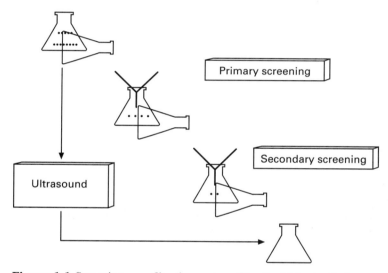

Figure 1.1 Screening as a filtration system. The liquid in the flasks represents the whole population being screened. The black dots in the liquid represent truly abnormal cases. The first screening examination (primary screening) is represented by the first filtration. It is hoped that most of the abnormal cases will be identified at this stage but some may not. Further examinations (referred to as secondary, tertiary, etc. screening) will filter out the remaining cases and must do so at a stage in the diseases' natural history which confers some treatment or outcome advantage. In this diagram there is a clear suggestion that ultrasound screening *may* be such an improvement on clinical tests – that one test may be enough and that secondary etc. screening may become a thing of the past. The place of ultrasound in DDH screening is yet to be defined but the matter will be discussed further in Chapter 6.

abnormality for which screening has been highly effective. Usually, the screening test for a disease is much less accurate and this is certainly so in DDH. It may therefore be necessary to reapply the same or other tests at a later stage.

Timing of screening

The earlier DDH is detected the easier the treatment, the more effective the treatment, and the greater the likelihood that surgery can be avoided.

A schematic illustration of the borderline between the surgical and non-surgical management of DDH is shown in Figure 1.2. As a general rule, the later the disease is detected the greater the chance that surgery will be required for the reduction and stabilisation of the affected hip. Many surgeons believe that if the disease is detected in the first 4–6 months there is a reasonable chance that surgery can be avoided and that the outcome will be excellent (not an unanimous view). The treatment of 'late' DDH will be discussed in Chapter 2.

This is looked at in another way in Figure 1.3, as a timeline. There is a critical point after which surgical methods are more likely to be required. This point is not, however, well defined.

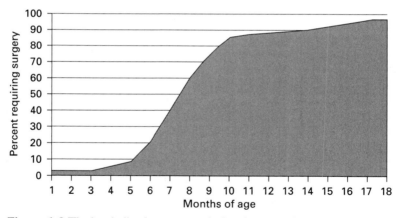

Figure 1.2 The borderline between surgical and non-surgical treatment. Surgical cases are shown in shading and non-operative cases by horizontal lines. The graph *only* shows the relationship between the time of detection and the chance of requiring surgical treatment For example, a case detected in the first 3 months has a very small chance of needing surgery but this chance increases rapidly between 5 and 10 months. A child presenting after walking has started is very likely to require surgery. *Note*: This graph does not represent the relative numbers of operative versus non-operative cases because the vast majority of cases are detected early and treated satisfactorily by simple splintage.

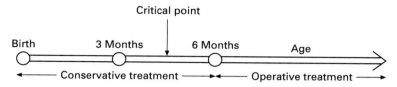

Figure 1.3 Timeline of the first year of life. Demonstration of the point in time when it becomes likely that operative treatment is needed. This is the 'Critical point'.

Because screening is an epidemiological concept it is necessary to discuss briefly the fundamental principles of screening. For many readers of this book this will not be of great interest and these principles are regarded as 'dry' by most clinicians. For this reason, some aspects will be discussed later in this chapter. It is important to have a definition and to understand the ideal circumstances for screening, because only by doing so will it be possible for the reader to understand why the results of screening for DDH are not always as good as expected.

Definition

Screening is one of the methods of disease prevention. It is the term applied to the detection of disease in an early presymptomatic stage. It was originally applied to infectious disease and perhaps the earliest and most well known example is the use of mass radiography for the detection of pulmonary tuberculosis. Later, particularly in developed countries, various other diseases such as phenylketonuria became the subject of intensive and successful screening programmes. Current screening programmes are directed at degenerative and neoplastic disorders but the future may hold great hope for those suffering from genetically transmitted diseases because screening techniques are now also applied to people who are potential carriers of disease.

Screening has been defined in several ways, but one accepted definition is that of Wilson in 1963:

> Screening is the use of quick and only
> approximate tests or examinations to
> differentiate those who *probably* have some
> disorder (especially a latent one) from those
> who *probably* do not.

The same author describes the ideal situation in which a screening test could be applied:

> A potentially serious condition is highly prevalent among the population and it exists in a latent or presymptomatic stage, the detection of which, if left to ordinary clinical methods, would require a high expenditure of medical manpower. A relatively simple test exists which, without the need for preliminary medical examination, will reveal those who probably have the condition. Those who are 'positive' on screening are physically examined and further tests are carried out. Finally, those with a positive diagnosis are treated, since the disease is curable.

Such ideal situations are rarely met in clinical practice. What, therefore, are the individual features which should help in the decision as to whether a proposed scheme of screening is appropriate? These factors relate to the disease and to the test.

The disease must be significant, have a reasonable incidence, be treatable and have treatment readily available. The test should be simple, reliable, acceptable to the parents as well as the baby and cheap.

There are two facts relating to the natural history of DDH which makes screening difficult. Firstly, as many as 20 babies in every 1000 births have unstable hips but 90% of these will stabilise themselves spontaneously. It is not possible to predict which 10% of these hips will remain unstable. Many have pondered on why this is so. The likely answer is provided in the anatomical study of Ralis and McKibbin, who showed that the hip is at its most unstable at the time of birth (being much more stable *in utero* and in the postnatal period). This is because early in gestation the acetabulum starts off as a complete sphere. A cleavage in the mesoderm develops which is to become the hip joint. In the development of the hip joint, the total spherical enclosure of the femoral head gets less and less to allow movement and therefore gets shallower during development. At about 38 weeks of gestation it is at its shallowest and it then becomes deeper again in the postnatal period. The tightness of the uterus and the lack of freedom of movement of the legs *in utero* in the later stages of pregnancy are aetiological factors in DDH. This of course fits in with the well known postnatal adverse environmental 'causes' of DDH; e.g. tight swaddling and splintage in extension, which was practised fairly widely by the Laplanders (see Chapter 2) in Northern Sweden. This may offer an explanation of the fact that the incidence of DDH is less in prematurely born babies. Another explanation is that in these babies there is no uterine constriction, i.e. they are fully mobile *in utero* with no compression by the uterus.

Secondly, there are hips which appear to be stable at birth even when examined by very experienced examiners which later can be shown to have DDH.

Two other approximate definitions are necessary at this stage, although the formulae for their calculation will be discussed later for those who need to know them.

The sensitivity of a test is the percentage accuracy of the test in detecting all the truly abnormal cases.

The specificity of a test is the percentage accuracy of the test in excluding the truly normal cases from further consideration.

Secondary screening

Sometimes it is necessary to carry out a screening test (which may or may not be the same test) at a later date. This is called *secondary screening* and it is particularly important when it is known that the first or primary test will not detect all the abnormal cases.

Selective screening

When only a proportion of the population at risk receives the test, this is known as *selective screening*. Special selection criteria are defined to select the patients who have a particular risk of having the disease.

The predictive value of a test is the percentage of the cases which were identified as probably having the disease who are later found truly to have had the disease and thus truly required treatment.

From this it can be seen that a test for DDH may be very sensitive (and it would need to be, because in a population say of 5000 births only one case needs be missed to give a 10% failure rate). However to identify 100% (which may only be 10 cases), the test has to question the normality of a further 100 or so cases, the predictive value would be low (at 10%) and thus the test would be far less acceptable.

Further consideration of
the epidemiology of screening

The efficiency of screening

A screening programme needs to be continually monitored, but *at the outset* it is most important to be certain that the aforementioned criteria are satisfied. If the criteria are satisfied, the validity of the test which will be used should be measured. This is done by measuring the 'sensitivity' and 'specificity' and 'predictive value' of the test. These parameters have a very specific meaning and method of measurement.

Validity

This is a measurement of the performance of a test compared with a reference test which is know to be 100% correct. The validity is made up of two components: (i) sensitivity and (ii) specificity.

Sensitivity

This is a measurement of the ability of a test to detect a high proportion of true cases, i.e. a sensitive test will detect a high proportion of truly abnormal patients. It is defined according to this formula:

$$\text{Sensitivity} = \frac{\text{True positives}}{\text{True positives + false negatives}} = \frac{\text{Correctly identified true positives}}{\text{Total true positives}}$$

A sensitivity of 1.0 (often referred to in percentage terms as 100%) means that the test will detect *all* the abnormal cases. In the above formula the term 'total true positives' is made up of (i) the correctly identified true positives and (ii) the abnormal cases which the test failed to identify (false negatives).

Specificity

This is a measurement of the ability of a test to reject the false positives, i.e. a specific test will have very few false positives. It is defined according to this formula:

$$\text{Specificity} = \frac{\text{True negatives}}{\text{True negatives + false positives}} = \frac{\text{Correctly identified true negatives}}{\text{Total true negatives}}$$

i.e. a specificity of 1.0 (or 100%) means the test will reject all the truly negative cases. In the above formula the 'total true negatives' are made up of (i) correctly identified true negatives and (ii) false positives.

The balance between sensitivity and specificity will vary according to the particular disease in question, e.g. if diagnostic criteria are stringent then there will be few false positives, but the test will be insensitive. Alternatively, if the criteria are relaxed, there may be a lot of false positives but the test will be less specific.

The predictive value

When a screening test is applied there will be a *yield* of what are considered to be abnormal cases. Some of these cases will be truly abnormal (let these = a), and some will on further testing be shown to be normal (let this number = b). The predictive value for a positive test is therefore as follows:

$$\text{Predictive value} = \frac{a}{a + b}$$

which represents the likelihood of a patient with a positive test actually having the disease. The predictive value tends to decrease when the population is large and the prevalence of the disease low. The number of false positives is often too high to be acceptable, e.g. screening for carcinoma of the breast using palpation and mammography.

The importance of false positive results

This is well illustrated in Figure 1.4. The less accurate the test is the more false positives will be diagnosed. This type of analysis (called ROC for Receiver Operated Characteristic) is really an illustration of the relationship between sensitivity and specificity and was first used in the assessment of the decision-making behaviour of radar operators, and has been adapted to assess screening tests.

False positives are inevitable although undesirable. The concept of trade off between sensitivity and specificity is a very real one. The same low threshold that makes a test highly sensitive (and therefore able to detect 100% of abnormal cases) also makes it likely that an increasing number will be falsely thought to have the condition (low specificity).

The importance of false negative results

A false negative result is what is often referred to as a missed case. It is the ultimate failure criterion in a screening event. The nearer the false negative rate is to the expected number of cases in an unscreened population,

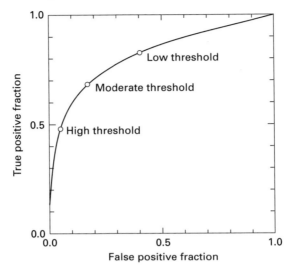

Figure 1.4 ROC curve illustrating the inevitable trade off between sensitivity and specificity. The y axis can be considered to be a measure of the sensitivity of the test, i.e. the nearer to the value of 1 the more the test approaches 100% sensitivity. The x axis can be considered to be a measure of specificity, i.e. the nearer the value is to 1 the more the test approaches 100% specificity. (Note the reversal of the direction of the y axis on the right!) (After Mant and Fowler, 1990, with permission.)

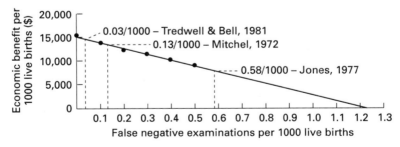

Figure 1.5 The relationship between economic benefit and false negative screening. The x axis shows the false negative results, i.e. so-called missed cases. The further along the x axis one goes the less sensitive the test. If the testing is highly sensitive then the false negatives will approach zero and at this point the cost effectiveness is greatest. (After Treadwell, 1990, with permission.)

the less effective the screening programme. In Figure 1.5. this is shown in the form of cost effectiveness, but the word 'cost' is not necessary in terms of the principles of screening.

Summary

In this chapter, the following will have been learned:

1. To define screening
2. To describe the ideal situation for screening in terms of the disease and the test.
3. To explain to parents what is meant by using an analogy with a filtration system.
4. That the primary screening tests are not perfect and that is why further examinations are needed at a later date (secondary screening).

Screening is not an easy concept to grasp but you should now be in a position to understand it and be able to give a 'lay' explanation without using technical jargon.

Further reading

Davies, S.J. and Walker, G. (1984). Problems in the early recognition of hip dysplasia. *J. Bone Joint Surg.*, **66B**, 479–484.

Ilfeld, F.W. and Westin, G.W. (1980). 'Missed' or late-diagnosed congenital dislocation of the hip. A clinical entity. *Isr. J. Med. Sci.*, **16**, 260–266.

McKeon, T. and Lowe, C.R. (1966). *An Introduction to Social Medicine.* Oxford: Blackwell.

Ralis, Z.A. and McKillin, B. (1973). Changes in shape of the human hip joint during its development and their relation to its stability. *J. Bone Joint Surg.*, **55B**, 780–785.

Rose, G. and Barker, D.J.P. (1986) *Epidemiology for the Uninitiated*, 2nd edn. London: BMJ Publishing Group.

Wilson, J.M.G. (1963). Multiple screening. *Lancet*, **2**, 51–54.

2

The treatment of 'missed' or 'late' DDH

Before discussing treatment, the influence of environmental factors during the early months of life will be discussed briefly.

Adverse postnatal influences

It was mentioned in Chapter 1 that there is very good evidence for believing that cramped circumstances *in utero* predispose to developmental dysplasia of the hip. It is well recognised that oligohydramnios and any signs of moulding in the baby are risk factors. The implication is quite clear – that pressure from the uterus on the baby so limiting the free movement of the lower limbs is a contributory factor to the development of DDH. As was also pointed out in Chapter 1, the acetabulum is at its shallowest at about 38 weeks of development but the increase of the acetabular depth in the early months of life is not particularly rapid and from an anatomical point of view the hip remains vulnerable.

The ideal situation for the hip both *in utero* and in the postnatal period is that it has freedom of movement and that easy abduction is allowed. Some would argue that in the postnatal period abduction is a very desirable position and should be aimed at in any prevention programme for DDH. The most persuasive argument for this in population terms is the interesting work of Klisic in Belgrade (Klisic *et al.*, 1988). From 1973 he introduced 'baby packages' free of charge which were distributed widely – these packages contained the equivalent of a double towel nappy or diaper. Soft abduction pants were worn over the diapers. It appears from his figures that in population terms it halved the number of late presentations from DDH and drastically decreased the number of operations required. It is not clear, with the subsequent developments in that part of the world, what has happened since that time, but the information provided is extremely interesting from an epidemiological aspect.

As will be discussed later, it is unclear why this condition of DDH appears to have increased despite the introduction of screening programmes. One explanation is based upon the fact that the true incidence of the condition has increased and if that is so one can only speculate as to the reason. Some research workers have speculated that the hormonal influences of the use of the pill as a contraceptive might have some relevance but it is my view that it is much more likely that the introduction of disposable nappies has been a much greater adverse influence. Such nappies do of course have considerable advantages but one of the disadvantages is that they are designed not to cause abduction of the hips. Unfortunately this problem will probably not be investigated satisfactorily, because returning to the traditional towelling nappies would simply be unacceptable to the population as a whole, even on an experimental basis.

Nursing habits

The highest incidences of DDH have been reported in the Laps and certain American Indians. This was well reviewed by Salter in 1968. There is known to be a high incidence in the Navajo Indians in Arizona. They lace their infants to cradle boards with the legs fully extended. This both immobilises the legs and put the hips under a certain amount of stress. It is also known that the Laplanders similarly treat their infants leading to an extremely high rate of late DDH.

In the North Canadian Indians where the mothers have traditionally carried their infants on their backs strapped to a cradle board with the legs extended and adducted, the frequency of DDH discovered late was some ten times as high when a cradle board is used. Among just over 2000 children carried in this way there were 250 cases of DDH (12.3%), compared to only 17 cases among 1347 (1.2%) when the cradle board was not used.

Similarly among the Laps, who are a small ethnic and nomadic group of people inhabiting the northern parts of Sweden, they kept their children in a structure called a 'Komsion' which was a boat-shaped cot covered with fur. In this cot the child's legs were wrapped up and totally extended and adducted. The study of Melbin showed that in a population of 813 children the frequency of late DDH was 2.5%.

In the case of the North Canadian Indians, Salter managed to persuade some to give up the use of the board but the ones who did not give up the board were persuaded to shorten the bag by half. This allowed the children to hyperflex the hip and knee joints and the frequency of late DDH decreased by some tenfold.

From these historical studies there can be little doubt that it is possible, *providing the basic tendency is present*, for babies' hips to be very adversely affected by the postnatal environment. It is almost certainly a combination of genetic tendency and environmental precipitation or aggravation.

On the other hand, the incidence of late DDH in African babies is so low that the disease is a rarity. African babies are traditionally carried on their mother's back with the legs widely abducted and it is inviting to attribute the rarity of the disease to this particular environmental nursing habit. It has, however, been shown by Skirving and Scadden (1979) that the African acetabulum is intrinsically deeper than the European acetabulum.

What are the lessons to be learned?

There are no nursing habits currently used in the UK which approximate to those described above (with the possible exception of the Welsh Shawl – but this is only mildly restrictive compared with the other methods mentioned). Nevertheless there is a lesson to be learned and the lesson is this, that the babies' hips like to be freely mobile and certainly the position of abduction is preferable to any adduction. There is some circumstantial evidence that swaddling babies can have an adverse influence, and many use this reason to explain the higher incidence of DDH in babies born in the winter time and of course the higher incidence in the left hip which is usually the uppermost hip when a baby lies on its side, the hip then falling into a natural position of adduction.

Perhaps therefore parents should be advised to do the following:

1. To allow free movement of the hips.
2. To position the baby in such a way that the hips will be more likely to be abducted than adducted, i.e. with current fears regarding the sudden infant death syndrome the prone position has been forbidden but the parents have a choice between the side position and the supine position and perhaps we should be persuading them to use the latter method.

Treatment of the 'missed' case

Why is it necessary to include this subject in a book which is designed to help in the prevention of this precise circumstance? There are several reasons. Firstly, we must continually remind ourselves that the penalty for lack of vigilance and attention to detail may lead to this penalty, which is a very heavy one for the child and the parents and the screeners. Secondly, it is necessary to discuss the concept of blame which is implicit in the term 'missed'. Many experienced examiners had been aware of cases which they had considered to be normal on neonatal examination, only to be later diagnosed as 'late DDH'. There are two important publications drawing attention to the possibility that the dislocation may develop over the months after the neonatal examination (referred to in the USA as the 'Ifield Phenomenon'). The first of these publications in 1980 by Ifield and Westin describes 10 cases in which 'physicians may be blamed erroneously for failure to diagnose DDH, and concludes that the possibility of delayed dislocation of the hip needs further study and its recognition is important for the medical and legal professions. The same phenomenon was clinically recognised in the UK in 1984 by Davies and Walker and more recent ultrasound studies prove the fact that hips can appear to be normal on clinical examination and yet be structurally abnormal.

> **Tip**
>
> **You may very well be confronted with the following question: is it possible to confirm, on the basis of a clinical examination alone, that a baby's hips are normal? The answer is 'no'. There is good evidence that even the most experienced examiners have failed to detect any abnormality in hips which have later been shown to be abnormal.**
>
> **However this exceptional situation must not be allowed to cloud the fact that in the vast majority of cases, if there is an abnormality present which matters, then there is a good chance it will be detected.**

The treatment of late DDH does depend on several factors, but in general the earlier the diagnosis is made the easier the treatment and the less likely surgery will be required (see Figures 1.2 and 1.3).

> **Tip**
>
> **It is very important that parents grasp the concept that the earlier treatment begins the more effective that treatment is.**

Once the diagnosis of the 'late' case is confirmed by X-ray, the parents will have a whole series of questions, the answers to which have to be provided whilst they are in a very emotional state. This must be done gently, sensitively but with complete honesty, and in my own practice I supplement the consultation with a short written explanation, because much of what is said is not understood at that time. Figures 2.1 and 2.2 demonstrate such a case.

Tip

Explanation for Parents
Your baby has been diagnosed as having developmental dysplasia of the hip. This used to be called CDH – congenital dislocation of the hip. Although you will feel very disappointed, it is much better diagnosed than left undetected and although treatment is necessary there is every chance now that your baby will have a normal hip.

In order to make the hip normal:

1. **Baby will have to come into hospital. (You may stay with baby the whole time.)**
2. **Baby's hip tissue will have to be loosened by a short period of traction – this is not painful and will not worry baby, although the look of it might be upsetting to you!**
3. **An examination is carried out under anaesthesia and through a pinhole incision tight muscles in the groin will be released and dye will be placed into the joint and X-rays taken. This is called an arthrogram and it is a way of being certain that the ball of the hip is in a correct position in the socket.**
4. **If there is some tissue stopping the hip going back (reducing) then an operation is carried out.**
5. **The surgeon will then assess whether or not a stabilising operation is necessary about 6 weeks later. This may be an operation to cut the bone and change its shape by inserting a small plate.**
6. **Finally the development of the socket (the acetabulum) will be monitored by X-ray over the next few years and if it does not develop properly an operation called an acetabuloplasty or pelvic osteotomy will be needed to complete the reconstruction.**

Remember the chances are that just the one procedure followed by several months in a cast is needed, but it is important for you to realise that if one or more other procedures are necessary it is not because something has gone wrong.

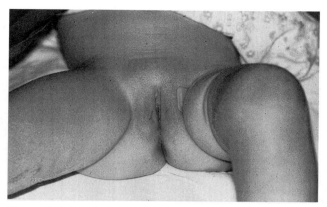

Figure 2.1 A typical case of a girl aged 1 year who is just starting to walk but limps and presents with a short leg, limitation of abduction and telescoping of the left hip.

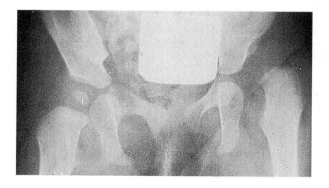

Figure 2.2 Radiograph of the girl in Figure 2.1, showing the dislocated left hip.

The principles of treatment

These are three:

1. Early detection
2. Reduction
3. Stabilisation.

Early detection

Generally, the earlier the disease is detected the better the outcome and the less the treatment required. For example, many centres do not treat unstable hips for the first 2 weeks of life on the basis that the majority of them will correct themselves and that splintage may harm them. Others (I include myself in this group) believe that with simple abduction splintage it is best to treat them all and this can be done without complication.

Even if we could be certain that screening would always detect every single potential late case, early detection does *not invariably* lead to a quick and successful outcome.

Reduction

When the condition does not present in the neonatal period it is increasingly detected at the child surveillance examination at the 6- or 8-month stage, but if not then at the time of walking which is usually at just beyond the 1-year stage. The details of management will vary from centre to centre but the principles will be the same. This may be either:

A. Closed
or
B. Open

The younger the patient the more likely closed reduction will be possible. (Some surgeons feel that if open reduction is necessary they prefer to wait until the baby is about 1 year old and leave the hip untreated in the interim period. This was based on fear of avascular necrosis and the size of the baby. With modern anaesthesia, however, and with evidence accumulating that avascular necrosis is not a particular age-related risk, many surgeons now question that traditional approach.)

The importance of gentleness cannot be overstated. In the days of Lorenz this fact had not been appreciated and therefore reduction could be quite rough. The danger is that in reducing the hip its delicate blood supply will be damaged resulting in a disease known as avascular necrosis of the femoral head. There are varying degrees of severity of this condition but in the more severe grades its effect on the child can be worse than the dislocated hip and therefore it is a condition very much to be avoided. In order to make sure no force is used several precautionary measures are taken. Firstly, there is a period of traction which as long as it is not used as a method of reduction, i.e. with the feet together and without abduction of the hips, is a simple harmless way of stretching the tissues. Secondly, because the adductors are likely to be tight, especially in abduction, they should be tenotomised before reduction and this can be done using a percutaneous technique. Thirdly, an arthrogram at the time of reduction proves concentricity and prevents the damage that may be caused by abducting the hip against an obstructive factor such as an inturned limbus. In this respect, one refers to 'the gentleness of the knife', an expression often used by one of the great British founders of paediatric orthopaedics, Mr Arthur Eyre-Brook of Bristol. One cannot overemphasise the fact that the careful cutting of tissue which is causing an obstruction is far less forceful than using a lever the length of a baby's leg in order to 'manipulate' a hip. The forces generated by such a lever are enormous.

If the hip cannot be safely, gently and concentrically reduced then an open reduction should be carried out. The commonest approach is anteriorly usually with a skin incision that is parallel to the groin and gives a good cosmetic result. The hip is exposed and all obstructive factors are removed allowing a concentric reduction.

Stabilisation

At this time the surgeon will carefully assess the position of the leg which allows the head of the femur to be deeply contained within the acetabulum. The surgeon may *plan* further surgery at this stage although it is not usually carried out for 6 weeks. The commonest stabilising operation is the rotation varus osteotomy of the femur (Figure 2.3). The osteotomy is held by a form of internal fixation such as the Coventry screw plate.

Sometimes a pelvic osteotomy (Salter) is used as an alternative, but it has the disadvantage that it is difficult to do under 18 months of age.

Once the toddler is walking the hip is checked out regularly both clinically and radiographically and an assessment is made of acetabular development. If this is unsatisfactory, then further surgery will be recommended to either re-orientate the acetabulum so that it gives better femoral head cover, as in the Salter osteotomy (Figure 2.4), or the acetabulum is altered in shape by re-orientating its roof, as in various acetabuloplasties, e.g. Pemberton's (Figure 2.5), Parker's, Trevor's. If there is a femoral plate to remove then this is best delayed until it is known whether or not acetabular surgery is going to be required. The plate can then easily be removed at the same time as the acetabular surgery, thus allowing the parents to perceive this all as one procedure.

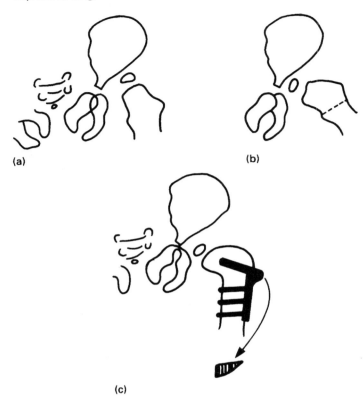

Figure 2.3 Diagrams illustrating: (a) a dysplastic subluxating hip; (b) concentric reduction in abduction and internal rotation; (c) osteotomy of the femur with Coventry screw plate fixation maintaining the hip as in (b) but enabling the legs to function in the normal walking position.

In my experience it is quite rare to require acetabular surgery if *early* concentric reduction is established and maintained.

It is usual for the child to be followed up until puberty.

Genetic counselling

Every time a baby is diagnosed as having a true DDH, whether it is on ultrasound or X-ray, the baby is identified as possessing some of the genetic material relating to the risk of this condition and therefore by implication there may be:

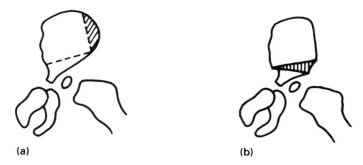

(a) (b)

Figure 2.4 The Salter osteotomy for changing the orientation of the acetabulum. (a) The position of the pelvic osteotomy and site of the graft is shown (hatched). (b) The acetabulum has been rotated downwards and forwards – the graft inserted and held in position by a metal wire which is removed when the bone has healed.

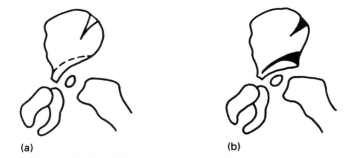

(a) (b)

Figure 2.5 The Pemberton osteotomy. (a) The position of the curved osteotomy extending down to the triradiate cartilage of the acetabulum. (b) Graft inserted changing the shape of the acetabulum from a saucer to a cup.

Tip

Genetic Counselling
Whilst there is no need to refer these parents to special genetic clinics which are now available in large hospitals, it is important to have available the facts quoted in the text because not only may you be asked but you should in a most careful way indicate the slight but definite increased risk for future siblings and the need for ultrasound scanning in such babies.

1. Further risk for the parents in terms of future births.
2. Risks for when the baby is grown up as a risk passed on to his/her children.
3. Implications for other members of the family, i.e. siblings of the baby.

The genetic predisposition for DDH is at least twofold:

1. The laxity of the tissues (probably collagen related and may well be related to the proportion of collagen type 3 present in the joint capsule).
2. Acetabular dysplasia.

If the individual affected is a child, then siblings of that child have a risk of 6% of developing the disease.

Tip

Genetic advice for the baby
It is very important that parents grasp the concept that the earlier treatment begins the more effective that treatment is. Although it is likely to be at least 16 years away, someone, perhaps the immediate mother or father, must be made aware of the increased risk for the grandchildren
It is, of course, very important not to frighten the patients with these details and always to emphasise that the whole purpose of warning them is that this is a totally curable condition which is best diagnosed early. It is never a factor to be taken into account in decisions about whether to have children.

If the individual affected is a parent then the first child of that parent has a risk of 12% of developing the disease, and if that first child does in fact develop the disease then the risk for the second child is approximately 36%.

Second-degree relatives such as cousins, nieces, nephews, etc., do have some increased risk but it is slight and estimated to be less than 1% (these figures are quoted from Harper, 1993).

Further reading

Berman, L. and Klenerman, L. (1986). Ultrasound screening for hip abnormalities: preliminary findings in 1001 neonates. *Br. Med. J. [Clin. Res.]*, **293**, 719–722.
Bower, C., Stanley, F.J., Morgan, B., Slattery, H. and Stanton, C. (1989).

Screening for congenital dislocation of the hip by child-health nurses in Western Australia. *Med. J. Aust.*, **150**, 61–65.

Mant, D. and Fowler, G. (1990). Mass screening: theory and ethics. *Br. Med. J.*, **300**, 916–918.

Ralis, Z. and McKibbin, B. (1973). Changes in shape of the human hip joint during its development and their relation to its stability. *J. Bone Joint Surg.*, **55B**, 780–785.

References

Davies, S.J.M. and Walker, G. (1984). Problems in the early recognition of hip dysplasia. *J. Bone Joint Surg.*, **66B**, 479–484.

Harper, P.S. (1993). *Practical Genetic Counselling*. Oxford: Butterworth-Heinemann.

Ilfeld, F.W. and Westin, G.W. (1980). 'Missed' or late-diagnosed congenital dislocation of the hip. A clinical entity. *Isr. J. Med. Sci.*, **16**, 260–266.

Klisic, P., Zivanovic ,V. and Brdar, R. (1988). Effects of triple prevention of CDH, stimulated by distribution of 'baby packages'. *J. Pediatr. Orthop.*, **8**, 9–11.

Meltin, T. (1962). The children of Swedish nomad Lapps. A study of their health growth and development. *Acta. Paediatr. Scand.* [Suppl.] 131.

Salter, R.B. (1968). Etiology, pathogenesis and possible prevention of congenital dislocation of the hip. *Can. Med. Assoc. J.*, **98**, 933.

Skirving, A.P. and Scadden, W.J. (1979). The African neonatal hip and its immunity from congenital dislocation. *J. Bone Joint Surg.*, **61B**, 339–341.

3

The clinical tests – how to do them

There has been and there continues to be a great deal of confusion about the names of these tests and the precise method of performing them. The confusion has arisen for a variety of reasons, but the main problems have been related to the fact that the tests are not simple and therefore are not easy to learn from books. Perhaps just as important has been the simple fact that Ortolani published his description in Italian and much was lost in translation and therefore from the outset there was confusion over the term 'click' and the term 'clunk'.

Parts of this chapter will therefore inevitably be historical but I believe that it is important to enter into a discussion on this if only because the name *Ortolani* has become almost synonymous with *screening*. It must also be emphasised that it is difficult to teach a test which is essentially a three-dimensional manoeuvre by referring to two-dimensional diagrams. Although this was addressed by the introduction of a teaching aid called 'Baby Hippy' in the USA, it was not an accurate model in so far as it failed to give the right feel of the magnitude of the forces involved. The best method of learning these tests was to watch them being done or, failing that, to watch a film or video. The latter is in some ways preferable because the spectre of 20 learners descending on an unfortunate baby in order to experience the positive result has to be seen to be believed! This, almost certainly, is not in the baby's interest. I have observed many experienced examiners carrying out these tests and I can testify to the wide variation in technique used. This has been studied by Professor Mollan in Belfast (Mollan *et al.*, 1983) and observation of some of his video recordings of examinations confirmed that this variation in technique is geographically widespread.

Perhaps the most surprising thing about all this is that, at no stage, did any official body, and in particular The Standing Medical Advisory Committee and the Standing Nursing and Midwifery Advisory Committee, ever question the suitability of such tests in the process of screening. They made recommendations in their 1969 and 1986 reports which will be discussed later in this chapter, but they did not question the conventional wisdom despite the fact that at this time (1986) there was good evidence from an epidemiological point of view that screening (using clinical tests) was not effective. The 11-page booklet which was produced was widely distributed on a 'one off' basis, but a decade later it is difficult to find a copy. It has not yet been updated (June 1996) but a new version is long overdue. It is to be hoped that the effect of any future recommendations will be carefully audited on a national basis.

The Ortolani test – historical review

Many will feel that this eponym which has stuck, and cannot be unstuck, has allowed history to cheat two other workers – Piere Le Damaney and Roser – who should be recognised for their contribution.

Piere Le Damaney (1912)

The precise verbatim translation of the description (in French) is given in full in an article by J.W. Dickson. In this article Mr Dickson concludes: 'This seems so exactly the manoeuvre described by Barlow that a case may be made out for renaming, in Britain at least, either the Le Damaney test or possibly the Le Damaney/Barlow test.'

In many ways this Frenchman was half a century ahead of his time, for not only did he describe this test but he also carried out the first pilot study of screening a population of 1722 newborn babies, firstly in Rennes and then in Paris.

Roser (1864)

Roser in 1864 described loose hip joints in the newborn that could be luxated by adducting the thighs and then reduced by abduction, so there is great confusion about this test, starting from 1864, developing with Le Damaney in 1914 and culminating with Ortolani in 1948 and Barlow in 1962.

The Ortolani test – how to do it

The best way to learn this test is to watch it being done firstly on a video-recording by someone who has studied the process and is aware of the forces permitted and then to become an apprentice to the local screener.

Prerequisites

The following remarks apply to all clinical tests on the hips of newborns but are particularly applicable in the case of the Ortolani and Barlow tests because if these conditions do not apply then the test result will be at best unreliable and at worst misleading.

1. The baby must be warm and comfortable.
2. The baby must not be hungry or thirsty.
3. The baby must be on a firm flat surface. An examination trolley with a mattress on it is ideal but a cot with sides of any description is contra-indicated.
4. One of the parents should be present.
5. Sucking clear sterile fluid or the breast will often relax a tense baby.
6. The examiner should be comfortable (preferably sitting) at the foot end of the trolley facing the baby's perineum. The trolley should be fixed and the mattress should be firm and the height of the trolley should be approximately 3 feet (1 m).

If any of these conditions do not apply, particularly those relating to relaxation, it is best to abandon the examination and retry later.

Tip

In the real world of 'work-a-day' clinical practice these prerequisites will not always be present.
  You must strive to make them available to you.
  If, for some reason, you end up doing the examination in suboptimal conditions, it would be wise to record the fact so that the next examiner knows how much reliance to put on the result of the previous examination.

Preliminaries

The examiner should have by this stage taken a careful history so that it would be known whether or not this baby was in the high risk group. The examiner should also be satisfied that consent has been obtained. This will be discussed in Chapter 7, but suffice it to say that at this stage the best way of doing this, at present, is by issuing an information leaflet (see Figure 7.1) to all parents at prenatal assessment and classes and/or at delivery.

The general examination may identify risk factors in addition to those elicited in taking a history. The following may be seen:

1. Postural foot deformities
2. Plagiocephaly
3. Scoliosis
4. Syndromic facies
5. Asymmetrical skin folds
6. Prominent sacral dimple (debatable)
7. HMS (hypermobility syndrome).

The significance of asymmetrical skin folds

Many observers claim that this is of no significance whatsoever. For example, Barlow (1962) states that less than half the cases with dislocated hips had unequal skin folds and the great majority of those with asymmetrical skin folds were found to be normal. Also in a study of 500 healthy newborns, Palmen (1961) found that the medial skin folds were symmetrical in 40%, asymmetrical in 42% and were absent in 28%.

This may be true of thigh skin folds but the asymmetry of gluteal skin folds has not been studied so thoroughly and many observers (including the author) feel that asymmetry in this region may be of greater significance, especially if accompanied by asymmetry of the vulvar cleft. Buttock and adductor fold asymmetry can demonstrate an abnormal hip. Also as long ago as 1941, Chapple and Davidson reported that the inguinal fold on the side of displacement tends to conceal the vulva in the newborn placed in the supine position. Whilst there is now good evidence that asymmetry of inguinal folds in the 3–4 month-old infant (examined with the hips abducted) is highly significant (Figure 3.1), the importance of gluteal, buttock and inguinal fold asymmetry must still be regarded as being of unproved significance in the first few weeks of life.

The vast majority of babies who have unequal skin creases have normal hips.

The Ortolani test

Make sure all the above criteria are met.

1. Warm your hands.
2. With the hips flexed to a right angle, hold the lower femur gently so that the thumb is on the inner side and the fingers on the outer side.
3. Without using excessive force now abduct the hips.

Findings of inguinal folds

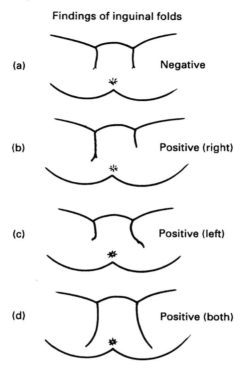

Figure 3.1 The inguinal folds on abduction in the 3- to 4-month-old baby, demonstrating the features that should be specifically looked for and recorded at this age: (a) short and symmetrical folds (normal); (b) asymmetry of folds, the longer fold on the right hip is positive; (c) asymmetry of folds, the longer fold on the left hip is positive; (d) symmetrical but long folds extending beyond the anus, right and left are positive. (Reproduced from Ando and Gotoh, 1990, with permission.)

4. A dislocated hip may (or may not) jump back into place with a clunk.

This is well demonstrated in a film made by Barlow and presented at a British Orthopaedic Association meeting in 1962. I have carefully studied a copy of the film (kindly loaned by Mr A. H. C. Ratliff of Bristol) and I am sure that the above description is what Barlow understood as the Ortolani test. In addition, I have also looked at a literal translation of Ortolani's original article (kindly provided by Mr Alan Fowler of Bridgend, who has made a very critical appraisal of the value of this test). In that translation it is quite clear that while the above stages were true at the outset, i.e. at the time of discovery of this phenomenon, Ortolani modified the test so that the thumb and the fingers had a more specific location:

> This sign is elicited with the patient lying down in supine position with the thighs in flexion and at right angles with the pelvis with a slight inward rotation, with the knees in flexion. A movement of abduction and external rotation of the thigh is produced holding the knee with the palm of the hand with the thumb in the inner side of the knee and producing, with the other fingers placed over the outer aspect of the thigh, pressure over the greater trochanter following a latero-medial direction.

It is quite clear, however, that there is no element of provocation in the Ortolani test.

The Barlow test

T. G. Barlow was an orthopaedic surgeon working at Hope Hospital in Salford. He started his investigations in 1957 and his work is well summarised in a review article written by him in 1962. He describes how he began to feel that the Ortolani test was inadequate and how he began to modify it:

> I began to modify the test until finally I was examining the children by placing each on its back with the legs towards the examiner, hips and knees flexed to the right angle and placing the middle finger of each hand over the child's greater trochanter, the flexed leg being contained in the palm of my hand and the thumb on the inner side of the thigh opposite the lesser trochanter.

Then with each leg held in 45 degrees of abduction, the middle finger of each hand is in turn pressed upon the greater trochanter to attempt to lift the femoral head into the acetabulum. If in so doing the femoral head does return to the acetabulum then the joint is dislocated, but, if no such movement occurs, the joint is not dislocated. Backward pressure is then exerted by the thumb on the inner side of the thigh, and, in some cases, the femoral head can be felt to slip backwards onto the posterior lip of the acetabulum. Such hips are not dislocated but unduly lax, and have been described as dislocatable ones.

This test has been and continues to be the subject of much controversy and this will be discussed later. However, now that the historical aspects of these eponymous tests have been outlined it is time to describe the combination of manoeuvres which can be recommended for routine use. It would, I believe, be historically accurate, but not exhaustively so, to call this the Roser–Le Damaney–Ortolani–Barlow test.

The practical test
(Roser–Le Damaney–Ortolani–Barlow test)

This is the test which the screeners should actually carry out. In carrying out the test, however, it is important to define the objectives. They are as follows:

1. To make general observations which may put the baby into a high risk group.
2. To diagnose dislocatable or dislocated hips.
3. To note the presence or absence of 'clicks'.
4. To record the range of abduction.

The description of this test by Palmen (1984) is excellent and is based upon his enormous personal experience. It is reproduced here almost verbatim.
Palmen describes three stages.

Stage 1: inspection

This consists of general observations referred to earlier.

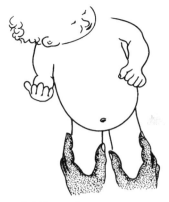

Figure 3.2 Roser/Le Damaney/Ortolani /Barlow Test: Stage 2 – the abduction test. This demonstrates the initial position of 90 degrees of flexion at the hip and knee joints. The hips are in a position of *add*uction.

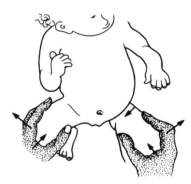

Figure 3.3 Roser/Le Damaney/Ortolani /Barlow Test: Stage 2. The arrows attempt to show the direction of the forces applied. The test consists of slow abduction with slight pressure in the direction of the arrows.

Stage 2: abduction

Take hold of the legs with your thumbs on the inside of the knees, and your fingers on the region of the greater trochanter. Keep the legs together completely adducted and stretched but without trying to force a possible restricted flexion of the hip and knee joints which is apparent in some newborns, especially during the first days. Check that the legs are of equal length. *Note*: straight back and symmetrical pelvis. Then flex the hip and knee joints 90 degrees (Figure 3.2).

Abduct slowly and carefully, with your whole hand, giving simultaneous slight pressure both in the direction of the thigh towards the joint and upwards with your fingers on the region of the greater trochanter (Figure 3.3).

If the femoral head is subluxated in the initial position you can feel a slight resistance when you have abducted about 45–60 degrees. Do not force the abduction if the child cannot relax. If you hold on with slight pressure the child will relax and you will gradually be able to continue abducting.

When you pass an abduction stage of 45–60 degrees you will distinctly feel the femoral head gliding or jumping into the centre of the acetabulum. If you then adduct again, pressing in the reverse direction, the femoral head will subluxate or dislocate again.

If stage 2 is negative go on to the next stage.

Stage 3: provocation of subluxation

In mild cases the femoral head may initially be at the centre of the joint at the preceding stage but then it can be made to subluxate by provocation.

From an initial position of 90 degrees of flexion and slight abduction (about 45 degrees), with your thumbs a little further towards the upper

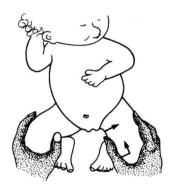

Figure 3.4 Roser/Le Damaney/Ortolani /Barlow Test: Stage 3. This is the stage of provocation illustrated by the examination of the left hip. The left hand supports the pelvis either in the way shown or more directly. The right hand is slowly abducted with slight pressure in the direction of the arrows.

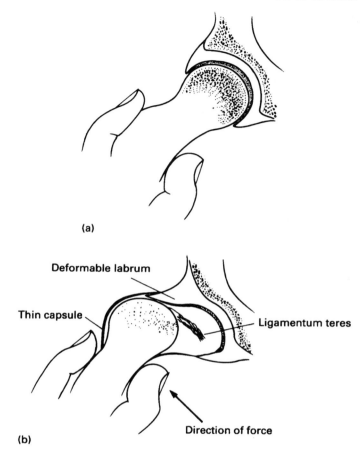

(a)

Deformable labrum

Thin capsule

Ligamentum teres

Direction of force

(b)

Figure 3.5 Roser/Le Damaney/Ortolani/Barlow Test: Stage 3. (a), (b) These cross-sectional diagrams show how the hip is posteriorly subluxated by the pressure applied through the thumb. The posterior capsule of the hip is a very thin and delicate structure at this age.

parts of the thighs, press slightly backwards – upwards with simultaneous slight adduction and inward rotation, as if the femoral head were to be subluxated (Figure 3.4). It is better to carry out this stage on one side at a time, while the other hand remains in the same position supporting the pelvis (Figure 3.5).

If instability is present, you will distinctly feel the femoral head being displaced backwards and upwards. Also reversing this stage, it can easily be moved back into the centre of the joint. The feeling of reduction will be more or less distinct.

In my experience these tests are less reliable the further away one gets from the neonatal period and although I have experience of these tests being positive at 3 months and 4 months of age, I believe this to be very uncommon and can see little point in persisting with such tests as a screening procedure beyond the 8-week stage. (However, some workers will consider this to be controversial.) It is much more important to embrace the concept of *secondary screening* than to insist that the process of primary screening has a 100% sensitivity. The most important test in this respect is the assessment of adductor tightness.

Tests depending on sounds or vibrations

Professor Mollan and his group have perfected the recording and interpretation of the noises which can be felt and heard on examining a baby's hips. They have marketed a device for the digital recording of data called 'The Belfast Hip Screener'. Although I have no experience of its use, the published results are encouraging and therefore it should be seriously considered in new screening programmes.

Test of restricted abduction

This is not a neonatal test and only becomes positive when the hip is dislocated and secondary shortening of the adductor muscles occurs. The fact that this test is of no value in the neonatal period is illustrated by the figures of Palmen (1984) (Table 3.1).

Table 3.1 Abduction of hips in the neonate

Abduction (degrees)	%
90–100	70
80	28
70	2

It is *the* test for secondary screening. It should therefore be used at the 8-week examination and every examination after that period including the 8-month examination. It is also an important sign before the 8-week stage but probably not as a screening test.

The baby must be relaxed and is placed in the same position used for the tests of hip instability. The hips are gently abducted and it should be possible to obtain almost 90 degrees of abduction, but force should not be used because it is not uncommon to demonstrate bilateral symmetrical limitation of abduction that is of no clinical or pathological significance.

Tip

Limited hip abduction
When this is discovered it is important to put the parents at ease by explaining to them that the chances are that this will not prove to be an abnormality in their child but further tests will be necessary to be sure.

You may also be greeted by the response 'why was this not detected earlier?'

Such a response must not generate resentment or irritation in the screener because it is a natural and reasonable question to ask and the answer to it is very simple: 'It was not present at the earlier examination, and the purpose of the present secondary screening examination is to search for signs such as these.'

Never be afraid to let the parents see the documentation of the previous abduction examination. With the newer parent-held neonatal record this information may already be in their possession.

Inguinal fold asymmetry

The work of Ando and Gotoh (1990) has to be regarded as very important in secondary screening for DDH. It gives us good reason to observe the inguinal fold symmetry at the time of measuring the degree of abduction. The findings on observation of the groins in abduction is illustrated in Figure 3.1. Whilst this phenomenon is very sensitive, i.e. all the abnormal cases on X-ray demonstrated the feature, it lacked specificity in that only 20–30% of those with this feature were truly abnormal.

The importance of 'secondary' screening

Unless or until a primary screening method is available with a sensitivity of almost 100%, it is always going to be essential to have in place the safety net of secondary screening.

Secondary screening in practice

The effectiveness of secondary screening has been demonstrated by Myles in an excellent study from Peterborough (Myles, 1990). He was able, with certain special arrangements for examination and referral, to reduce the number of late presenting cases from 2.18 per 1000 to 0.73 per 1000.

In most centres, however, secondary screening is likely to take place in such a way that it fits in with other paediatric examinations and immunisations. This means that in practice in the UK it will be done at 8 weeks and 8 months. It could be argued however that the ideal time would be at 3–4 months and this is supported by Myles' work.

The baby has to be comfortably relaxed and of course undressed. (I have seen abduction of the hips performed in varying degrees of undress!) The nappy should also be removed. Gluteal and inguinal skin creases should be observed with the legs together:

1. From the front with the legs extended.
2. From below with the adducted legs lifted vertically by the ankles.

The groin creases should then be observed with the legs in abduction and reference should be made to Figure 3.1.

Abduction should now be measured. The knees and hips are held at 90 degrees and the hips are gently abducted and an estimate is made of the degree of abduction, allocating a numerical value for the right and left sides. Force should not be used and as a simple test of this you can observe the capillary circulation in the thumbnail at the time of abduction (using only the thumb for this estimation of force). There should be no blanching of the thumb pulp of the examining hand.

Producing a numerical result is difficult and must be subject to a very wide observer error. It does, however, by forcing an estimate to be made for both hips, have the great advantage of concentrating the mind.

Interpretation of result

Of all the interpretations this is probably the most difficult. However it is probably the easiest to deal with, because on the basis of an abnormal result you are going to do one of three things:

1. Continue observation (unwise unless very experienced!).
2. Ultrasound (under 3 months).
3. X-ray (over 4 months). Great care must be taken in interpreting this

X-ray because it could lead the surgeon towards unnecessary treatment. The radiograph should be discussed with a radiologist who is familiar with the paper of Bowyer *et al.* (1985).

Unilateral limitation of abduction has to be taken very seriously because in this group there will be cases of subluxation or dislocation of the hip. However, the vast majority of cases will be examples of 'non-specific' abduction limitation which does not lead to dislocation but leads to the development of a normal hip. Is it possible to distinguish between these two groups by clinical methods? Probably not, but there are some important pointers which have been studied by Palmen (1961).

The importance of limited abduction in proven DDH is demonstrated in Table 3.2. In my experience, limited abduction is nearly always present in these circumstances and I have seen only four cases when it was not and these demonstrated *the very unusual* feature of a dislocatable hip beyond the 4-month stage.

Table 3.2 Hip abduction in 407 late diagnosed cases of DDH (Palmen, 1984)

Hip status	%
Abduction limited	80
Unstable	8
Unrecorded	12

What is a normal range of abduction? It should be at least 60 degrees in the first 6 months but any difference between the left and right side should be regarded as suspicious.

This whole question was carefully studied at Oswestry in 1985 by Bowyer *et al.* Most of the infants examined were 6 months or under and were referred because of limited abduction of the hip on routine examination. Cases of dislocation or subluxation were excluded from the study. These authors described a syndrome which has fairly definite features both clinically and radiographically and which has a benign outcome. The features are detailed below.

A baby of about 6 months is found to have limited abduction of one hip. The pelvis may appear oblique with tilting upwards on the side of the limited abduction. The gluteal folds may appear asymmetrical and the limb on the tight adductor side is apparently short. The radiograph may show a higher acetabular angle on the tight side, pelvic obliquity and a rotational deformation of the pelvis. This rotation makes the iliac blade look narrower on the anteroposterior X-ray. Most of these infants have plagiocephaly with the recessed side uppermost, some have transient scoliosis and other postural problems such as torticollis and foot deformities. What is the explanation of this benign phenomenon?

Palmen considers this to be a result of the baby lying in the 'habitually unilateral supine position', i.e. the baby is put to sleep in the supine position but sooner or later the trunk is turned usually to the right side allowing gravity to have an effect. The tight hip is the uppermost hip, the flattening of the head is on the uppermost side and the scoliosis, when present, is concave to the uppermost side.

It appears that only about 3% of cases of limited hip abduction will turn out to have a true DDH but it must be remembered that almost all cases of true DDH will have this sign.

The personnel requirement – who does it?

It is much easier to answer this question than to answer the real question of who should do it. At present it is done by a variety of health professionals and who knows how often by the parents themselves. This includes:

- Nurses and midwives.
- Paediatric senior house officers (SHOs).
- Senior paediatric medical staff.
- Physiotherapists.
- Health visitors.
- Orthopaedic staff.

The precise protocol will vary from district to district. Many places will not have a protocol and we know that 50% of health authorities have no individual nominated to be in charge of the screening programme (Jones *et al.*, 1989), as recommended by the Standing Medical Advisory Committee and the Standing Nursing and Midwifery Advisory Committee.

For purely practical reasons, this task has always fallen on the paediatric senior house officer (SHO) in the UK. This is not invariably the case, for there are specialised units where others have been trained, but this is certainly the typical situation.

Certain factors relating to the examiner have to be considered in detail:

1. Does he/she have sufficient time to devote to neonatal screening?

2. Are the duties of the SHO such that there are several things calling on his/her time simultaneously?
3. Has he/she had proper and specific training?
4. Has he/she ever felt the sensation of a subluxating or dislocating hip prior to starting the screening examinations?

Sadly, in the typical case none of these conditions apply and the inexperienced, untrained SHO with multiple calls upon his or her time is asked to carry out this examination.

It is known from certain published studies that the results of clinical screening can be extremely good (Hadlow, 1988, achieved a late DDH rate of 0.09 per 1000 births in a birth cohort of 20 000). A most instructive investigation of this precise issue was carried out by Krikler and Dwyer (1992). They compared two screening programmes in different hospitals of the same district. Both regimens used clinical tests only on newborn infants. In one group the screening was done by junior paediatric physicians (this usually means SHOs) and in the other group, senior physiotherapists carried out the examination under the supervision of an orthopaedic surgeon. To put a figure on it, it would appear that the physiotherapists were about three times as accurate as the junior medical paediatric doctors and the accuracy becomes increased if an interested consultant orthopaedic surgeon does the examination, as shown by the experiences of Krikler and Dwyer and Hadlow.

There is a clear relationship, therefore, between detection and expertise and these findings have to be taken into account in designing a screening programme. The findings, of course, refer to primary screening and the use of the Ortolani and Barlow tests.

The matter is quite different when it comes to secondary screening, perhaps at the 8-weeks stage where failure of the hips to fully abduct becomes a much more important physical sign and one which is far easier to interpret. This test may well be more accurate and easier to teach than tests of instability.

Primary hip screening should be done during the neonatal period and, ideally, it should be done by personnel who have been specifically trained to do it. It does not matter precisely which professional it is, but what does matter is that there is a bank of at least two such professionals (which would allow for holidays, etc.) and they must be fairly permanent members of staff. This almost automatically excludes paediatric SHOs from this task.

Perhaps the persons best suited to carry out this screening are paediatric physiotherapists but within the limitations described above. Midwives and health visitors are also suitable personnel to be trained for this important function. The efficiency of community nurses in this role has been shown in Western Australia by Bower *et al.* (1987). An editorial accompanying the article concluded that Bower 'had provided evidence that community nurses can perform screening for the presence of congenital dislocation of the hip at a highly competent level, possibly as good as or better than medical practitioners'.

In the general run of things, it does appear that the involvement of health visitors is usually at a later stage and that the involvement of midwives in neonatal hip examination is an extremely variable event. The problem of involving staff other than medical staff has always been the fear of litigation, and it was a very reasonable fear at the time when we did not fully understand the natural history of the disease.

Now that we have an understanding of the fact that a very abnormal hip may have no detectable physical signs at birth, the concept of 'fault' in 'missing' a DDH has largely gone. (It is important, however, not to allow the quotation of this fact to be used as a reason for complacency because it does not exclude the possibility that in any individual case an incompetent examination was carried out!)

References

Ando, M. and Gotoh, E. (1990). Significance of inguinal folds for diagnosis of congenital dislocation of the hip in infants aged three to four months. *J. Pediatr. Orthop.*, **10**, 331–334.

Barlow, T.G. (1962). Early diagnosis and treatment of congenital dislocation of the hip. *J. Bone Joint Surg.*, **44B**, 292–301.

Bower, C., Stanley, F.J. and Kricker, A. (1987). Congenital dislocation of the hip in Western Australia. A comparison of neonatally and postneonatally diagnosed cases. *Clin. Orthop. Rel. Res.*, 37–44.

Bowyer, F.M., Hoyle, M.D., McCall, I.W. and Evans, G.A. (1985). Radiological evaluation of asymmetrical limitation of hip abduction during the first year of life. *Br. J. Radiol.*, **58**, 935–939.

Chapple, C. and Davidson, T. (1941). A study of the relationship between foetal position and certain congenital deformities. *J. Paediatr.*, **18**, 483.

DHSS Report. (1986). Screening for the detection of congenital dislocation of the hip. Prepared by the Standing Medical Advisory Committee and The Standing Nursing and Midwifery Advisory Committee for the Secretaries of State for Social Services for Wales.

Jones, D.A., Beynon, D. and Littlepage, B.N.C. (1989). Audit of an official recommendation on screening for congenital dislocation of the hip. *B.*, **302**, 1435–1436.

Kernohan, W.G., Trainor, B.P., Haugh, P.E., Johnston, A.F. and Mollan, R.A. (1992). The Belfast hip screener: from infancy to maturity. *Ulster Med. J.*, **61**, 151–156.

Krikler, S.J. and Dwyer, N.S. (1992). Comparison of results of two approaches to hip screening in infants [see comments]. *J. Bone Joint Surg.*, **74**, 701–703.

Mollan, R.A.B., Bogues, B.A. and Cowie, G.H. (1983). A new aid in screening for congenital dislocation of the hip. *Health Visitor*, **56**, 285–287.

Myles, J.W. (1990). Secondary screening for congenital displacement of the hip. *J. Bone Joint Surg.*, **72**, 326–327.

Palmen, K. (1961). Preluxation of the hip joint. *Acta. Paed. Suppl.*, 129.

Palmen, K. (1984). Prevention of congenital dislocation of the hip. The Swedish experience of neonatal treatment of hip joint instability. *Acta. Orthop. Scand. Suppl.*, **208**, 1–107.

Further reading

Dickson, J.W. (1969). Piere Le Damaney on congenital dysplasia of the hip. *Proc. R. Soc. Med.*, **62**, 575–577.

Jones, D.A. (1977). An assessment of the value of examination of the hip in the newborn. *J. Bone. Joint. Surg.*, **59**, 318–322.

Jones, D.A. (1989). Importance of the clicking hip in screening for congenital dislocation of the hip [see comments]. *Lancet*, **i**, 599–601.

4

Child surveillance and the timing of screening

The timing of the screening test is of course of great importance. It is also of importance in a modern context that there is no re-duplication of effort, i.e. if a baby is being examined at certain times, it is important that the screening examination, particularly the secondary screening examinations, are carried out as part of examinations that would, in any event, have been carried out. The only disadvantage of this is in relationship to the personnel that are carrying out the test and that is that the ideal person for doing the screening test may not be the person who is scheduled to examine the patient for other reasons, e.g. immunisations and other child surveillance reasons. This has been discussed in the previous chapter.

Our aims in screening are clearly to detect the disease at the earliest possible stage so that treatment of a suitable nature can be instituted. Generally, it is hoped that the disease can be detected at a stage prior to the disease requiring surgery to cure it. In practice, this usually means finding the disease before the third or fourth month of life, although it has to be said that the screening process will of course continue until the child is ambulating normally. Every effort, therefore, should be made to detect all babies, certainly before the fourth month of life. This brings up the question as to whether every single case is abnormal by the fourth month of life and detectably so. In my experience, I would say that the abnormality is always detectable by that stage, particularly when the abnormality can be looked for using ultrasound and even X-ray.

Figure 1.3 illustrates the timing of detection in relation to the possible necessity for surgery, and although the critical point has been put at about the 3-month period, it remains a contentious issue and must not be adhered to rigidly. For example, babies as old as 2 years of age have had successful conservative treatment carried out on them after traction and an adductor tenotomy.

The timing of the tests – when should it be done?

In the UK this timing is determined by events which are unrelated to facts about the disease and are more related to when routine examinations are carried out for other reasons.

It is also important to think in terms of what is possible in practice. For example, it may be theoretically best for the hips to be examined say at 7 days, but for practical reasons the baby is never available to the examiner at that particular stage and therefore it would be impossible to examine a high proportion of cases and hence the screening progress will fail. The first 12 hours may not be the ideal time but it is the time which is best in terms of the screening process. In my opinion, however, I think it is the best time.

The timing of screening therefore depends on two factors:

1. The ideal time to detect the disease, i.e. this is one of the characteristics of the disease.
2. The ideal time to 'capture' the population.

Therefore since the vast majority of all births occur in hospital, the first 8 hours after birth represents the best time to examine the baby for DDH. This becomes especially true if the screening test depends upon some instrumentation which is only present in an institution, e.g. ultrasound. The next best time is at the 6–8-week examination because this is the point at which every child has to be examined for the purpose of the child surveillance programme. However, as discussed earlier, the examination to be carried out on the hips at this stage would be orientated more towards detecting failure of abduction than detecting hip instability.

Child surveillance

The term surveillance took on a new meaning when a new contract was offered to general practitioners (GPs) in the UK in 1990. The aim was that paediatric surveillance (Table 4.1) should find its proper place as an integral part of general practice and certain standards were set for accreditation for a GP to be on the Child Health Surveillance List. General practice was therefore set for an increasing role in the screening process and this was set to become a contractual issue. The idea, however, that general practice was the place for child health surveillance was not related

Table 4.1 Aims of a child health surveillance programme

To confirm normality and offer guidance on child growth and development
To pick up variations and deviations from normal development
To identify and follow up children with potentially handicapping conditions
To provide opportunities for parents to discuss their children's development and
health needs

to the change of contract directly for it was mooted some years ago in the
Court Report (Committee on Child Health Services, 1976). The guidelines
put forward by Curtis-Jenkins (1982) outline what a practice policy could
be for child surveillance:

> A commitment to the surveillance of children
> that is shared by the whole practice team.

> A clear outline of what the surveillance
> programme will entail and who will be doing
> what.

> A readily available up-to-date record of all
> children under 5 years in the practice.

> Keeping surveillance clinics separate from the
> routine care of sick children. (Failing to do
> this will result in confusion for parents about
> the role and function of child health
> surveillance clinics.)

> Continuous monitoring of performance: this
> can include a regular "spot check" of the
> practice team's target population register and
> review of non-attendance rates.

> Regular contact between doctors, health
> visitors, and other practice staff involved in
> organising pre-school examination.

In addition to these matters, it became obvious that the parents needed
recognition as true partners in the process of child health surveillance and
this became widely recognised, and it is now the case that most health
authorities have child medical records which are parent held. Some consideration has to be given as to how these parent-held records are dealt
with in busy screening clinics.

Children are examined at certain times and the surveillance key points are as follows:

- 6 weeks
- 8–10 months
- 18–24 months
- 36–39 months

The two periods which are particularly important in relation to screening for DDH are:

- The 6-week examination.
- The 8-month examination.

It would have been more ideal, as far as DDH is concerned, if there had also been a 3-month examination. The surveillance criteria allowed the GP to specifically target populations to provide facilities, equipment and time 'ring fenced' for these activities, also to go on specific training programmes and to be in a position to attempt to assess the effectiveness of child surveillance.

In addition to the examination, the importance of risk factors in the history must never be forgotten. Jones (1990) attempted to quantify the risk (Table 4.2).

Table 4.2 Quantification of the risk factors (after Jones, 1990)

Risk factor	Risk factor	Confidence limits
Family history	11.35	3.60–35.78
Clicking hip	10.36	6.04–10.78
Breech	5.49	2.38–12.64
Caesarean section	1.90	0.46–7.84
Worried examiner	7.91	2.91–21.49
Positive Ortolani test	90.94	63.8–129.5

Confidence intervals for $P = 0.05$, etc.

The timing of the examination

Clearly, the baby should be examined at the following times:

- During the first 24 hours.
- Prior to discharge from hospital (this examination will not take place if the child is discharged earlier).
- At home within the first few days of birth by the GP, clinical medical officer, midwife or health visitor.

- Subsequent occasions prior to the next formal screening examination.
- 8-month screening examination and 18–24-month observation of walking and gait. The latter is not in any way a screening examination, for it is merely an examination that may or may not detect problems in relation to DDH, which at this stage are highly likely to require surgery and are also highly likely to have presented in the normal way, complaining of symptoms.

These two examinations should be computer controlled, i.e. there should be a feedback method of recording whether or not the examinations have actually occurred (see Figure 9.2).

There will always be debate as to when screening should be carried out and whereas it was always thought that one could never examine a baby's hips too many times, there has been doubt brought upon that concept by the idea that it may be possible to damage a baby's hips by screening, particularly in using the Barlow test (Moore, 1989).

Gone, however, is the concept of blame in relationship to not being able to detect abnormal hips at birth. It was known from the work of Ifield and of Walker and Davies that it is possible for hips to be abnormal whilst appearing to be clinically normal around the neonatal period. This has now been proven time and time again by the application of ultrasound techniques, so as far as clinical screening is concerned it would appear that the examinations, particularly at the neonatal period and at 3 months, and certainly at 6–8 months, are essential if clinical screening only is to be relied upon.

These timings, however, may have to be considerably modified if ultrasound techniques come up to their expected accuracy.

We have concentrated upon these times as times of *examination*. However, it must not be forgotten that at the first opportunity, and at subsequent opportunities, the examiner must quickly go through his/her checklist of risk factors in order to pick out babies who may be at particular risk of this condition, and the documentation should reflect this.

References

Committee on Child Health Services (Court Report) (1976). *Fit for the Future*. (Cmnd. 6684). London: HMSO.

Curtis-Jenkins, G. (1982). The first five years of life. *Br. Med. J.*, **285**, 1175–1176.

Davies, S.J.M. and Walker, G. (1984). Problems in the early recognition of hip dysplasia. *J. Bone Joint Surg.*, **66B**, 479–484.

Ilfield, F.W., Westin, W.G. and Makin, M. (1986). Missed or developmental dislocation of the hip. *Clinical Orthopaedics*, **203**, 276–281.

Jones, D.A. (1990). MCh thesis. Screening for congenital dislocation of the hip. University of Wales.

Moore, F.H. (1989). Examining infants' hips – can it do harm? *J. Bone Joint Surg.*, **71B**, 4–5.

5

History and epidemiology – the results of clinical screening

This is a very important subject and the screener has to be very aware that screening is essentially an epidemiological concept and the results, unlike clinical studies, are based not simply on the cases that have been seen but upon the whole population. For example, a particular hospital in a large city publishes superb results for DDH screening, but when the results of late presenting DDH are analysed for that health district they may be found to be no better than the results for an unscreened population. It is the failure of clinicians to embrace this concept that has led to the many misunderstandings in the interpretation of the results of screening. What is the incidence of late presenting DDH in an *unscreened* population in the UK? It is impossible to study that question today (this very fact will be discussed in Chapter 7), but we do have data published as long ago as 1958.

The early studies

Births in Birmingham were studied between 1942 and 1952 (Record and Edwards, 1958), together with the details of late cases of DDH. This was a very careful study in which a lot of precautions were taken to make sure that all the cases within the birth population were included while all those outside it were excluded. The end result after examining over 200 000 births was a rate of late DDH of 0.65 cases per 1000 live births. Most observers would be slightly surprised by how low this figure is.

They noted the characteristics of the babies at highest risk, which were:

- Firstborn
- Girls
- Low birth weight
- Born in the winter months
- Positive family history.

The figure of 0.65 per 1000 was therefore considered to be the unscreened norm but it must be stated that there may be a variation in incidence even within the UK and, whilst the Midlands may have a low natural incidence, other areas such as Southampton may have a greater natural incidence (Wilkinson, 1987)

The second Birmingham study is equally as important because it is approximately the same population as previously studied in so far as time will ever stand still. There was no reason to believe that there had been any significant natural change. The study occurred between 1974 and 1983, neonatal screening having been introduced in November 1966 (Knox Armstrong and Lancashire, 1987).

The results not only showed that the incidence of cases requiring in-patient treatment had not declined but also indicated that the performance of the tests was poor with a sensitivity of only 33%. They also concluded that little thought had been given to quality control or measurement of the effectiveness of the system.

Later studies

In Southampton, 178 cases born between 1965 and 1978 were studied. Catford *et al.* (1982) showed that over this period the incidence of late cases had doubled. The very title of the paper caused alarm: 'Congenital hip dislocation; an increasing and still uncontrolled disability'. Six of the cases had risk factors identified and 76% of these were diagnosed in the first 2 months. However, the other 72 had only a 26% diagnosis rate in the same period. It was found that 55% of late cases presented because of parental concern, even though 90% of these had been the subject of several medical and nursing contacts (see Tip on page 2).

The most striking illustration of the conclusions of Catford *et al.* is shown in Figures 5.1 and 5.2.

Leck in 1986 directly compares screening for DDH with the criteria which every screening procedure should meet and concludes that the problems relate to false positives and false negatives. They found a very high number of false positives (ten times the number of true positives). About half of the cases were being missed but it is interesting that their approach was so scientific that they did not reach the simple conclusion that the examiners were failing to detect these cases but put forward the alternative possibility that the instability might have developed later. When they analysed the Bristol figures they concluded that the sensitivity of clinical neonatal screening was 66% with a specificity of 98%.

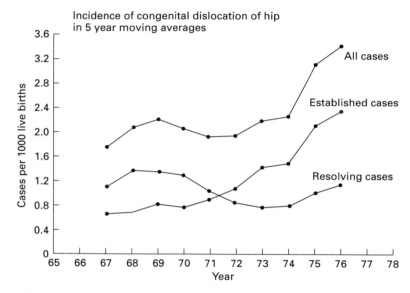

Figure 5.1 Graph illustrating the lack of a beneficial effect of screening for DDH which started in Southampton in the late 1960s; the incidence of established cases has gone up rather than down as might have been expected. (After Catford *et al.*, with permission.)

Clinical results versus epidemiological results

It must be remembered that clinical studies are usually carried out by clinicians who have a special interest in the disease of DDH and they tend to be reporting their experience of results of screening examinations. These are usually related to populations within a city but it must be remembered that some authors actually subdivide the city in such a way as only to report the results on babies that are born within their particular sector of the city. Studies such as the latter must be regarded with great suspicion and studies such as the former, which are far better, must also be interpreted with caution because it is important that those authors have ascertained the fact that no child has been referred to neighbouring areas for treatment of a condition which might have been missed in the screening process. Generally, these clinical studies are of high quality but they are always done by people with a special interest in the disease and therefore one can never tell whether the results obtained are due to the

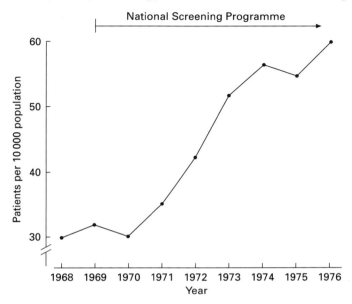

Figure 5.2 Graph demonstrating the overall apparent lack of any beneficial effect of screening in a population from prevalence of cases of DDH (0–4 years) admitted to National Health Service hospitals in England and Wales: 1968–76. (After Wilkinson, with permission.)

method which is used or whether they are due to some other more difficult to define effect, such as the enthusiasm of the author.

There have been several studies, the most outstanding of which is the study of Victor Hadlow who has obtained results from clinical screening which match the best results even using ultrasound (Hadlow, 1988). Authors of clinical studies such as these can usually give good reasons why other studies do not attain such good results. However, I do not know of any example where an author who has obtained extremely good results in one area, has then attempted to reproduce the method in another area (geographical area) where the supervising doctor has no particular special interest in the disease, for that is the ultimate test of any screening process.

Conclusion from the Swansea studies

These studies were designed to assess DDH screening in the light of the conditions laid down for screening in so far as they apply generally to any condition. These results were summarised in an Hunterian Lecture to the Royal College of Surgeons of England (Jones, 1994).

There are two studies which are particularly relevant to this chapter (Jones, 1990). I studied the figures available in the hospital activity analysis (HAA data) for Wales, the counties of Wales and in particular for West Glamorgan. West Glamorgan is one of the main centres of population in South Wales being one of the four fairly industrial counties of Gwent, South Glamorgan, Mid Glamorgan and West Glamorgan with a population at that time of 363 200 but providing health care to a population of rather more than this. Over the years 1979–1984 the birth rate was noted and during that time the screening process was fairly defined and fairly standard, with a paediatric senior house officer examining the baby within 24 hours of birth and then the baby being examined at about 6 weeks by the GP or clinical medical officer; most babies were also examined again at the age of 6 months. This programme of examination was not under any overall supervision, nor was there any record of its effectiveness or measurement of its effectiveness. The hospital activity analysis figures allowed me to make detailed observations of admission rates to hospital aged 4 weeks to 1 year and admission rates aged 1–4 years. Care was taken to be sure that admissions were identified on an individual basis so that the same patient was never counted twice, i.e. the number of admissions is going to be more than the number of patients. The conclusion reached was that between 1979 and 1984 there were 1.74 cases per thousand births of so-called late DDH and also that that figure could certainly not be an overestimate but there was still some possibility that it was an underestimate, i.e. perhaps not all cases were entered into the system.

In addition to looking at the West Glamorgan figures, I also looked at the figures for the whole of Wales. In all the major counties where referral patterns were well defined, a similar conclusion was reached and that conclusion can be stated as simply as this: that the effects of screening were neutral, i.e. screening did not appear to reduce the incidence of late DDH to a figure less than the natural history of the disease. Put more starkly, screening appeared to be pointless and, as will be discussed in a later chapter, there are negative effects of screening which are not generally known and understood.

As a result of this study, I carried out a further study which was a prospective clinical study in the year 1985/1986, and this was a simple study to try to determine the specificity and sensitivity of the simple clinical tests as carried out by fairly inexperienced paediatric senior house officers. The maternity services for the Swansea District of West Glamorgan were located at Morriston Hospital where the paediatric and orthopaedic departments were also located. The screening programme was allowed to go on in its normal way but, in addition to this, every baby who had any risk factor was sent for and re-examined by me personally within a week of the primary examination and, following that examination, the patient would be either discharged or referred for further investigation or treatment. During this period there were 3289 births and, out of these, 426 were referred for the special examination (12.9%). Of these, 51 were considered to have the possibility of an abnormality on clinical examination by the experienced observer, i.e. 1.55% of the birth cohort. Neonatal hip abnormalities were discovered in 4.5 per 1000 births by the paediatric senior house officer but this increased to 15.5 per 1000 births when 456 cases out of the birth cohort were re-examined on the basis of the babies having high risk factors. This indicated that the senior house officers were underdiagnosing the physical signs to the extent of 11 per 1000 births. The risk factors were analysed. Family history raises the risk by a factor of 11.35, a clicking hip increases the risk by a factor of 10.36, breech by 5.49, a caesarean section by 1.90 and the suspicion by the paediatric senior house officer in a way that he could not specifically define increased the risk by 7.91. This was the first attempt in the literature to try to quantify the increased risk on the basis of factors being present which put the baby into a special high risk group.

During the 12 months following this study, the high risk group became the subject of ultrasound screening as opposed to secondary expert screening. All screening tests must eventually be able to be done by a simple test which does not require the presence of a senior member of the department, for if it does that it fails to satisfy the criteria for a screening test.

Why has clinical screening been ineffective?

This question has been asked and answers have been attempted by many and several reasons have been put forward. Some of these have already been discussed, including the theory that the disease itself is getting more common. It has even been suggested that the process of screening itself has contributed to this increased incidence which is demonstrated most graphically by the paper of Catford *et al.* (1982) (Figure 5.1). Fred Moore of Cork is of the opinion that tests of provocation may be harmful and has collected data supporting this hypothesis.

The 1982 paper by John Catford, George Bennet and John Wilkinson from Southampton, 'Congenital hip dislocation: an increasing and uncontrolled disability', was a highly significant paper at a time when many institutions were publishing data to indicate that in a particular centre it was possible to almost eliminate the disease. The conclusion of this paper, which was written before audit was a buzzword, is worth quoting:

> Thus, neonatal screening appears to have failed to make a substantial impact on the morbidity of the disease, probably because of a combination of inherent difficulties in the neonatal screening test as well as failure in its proper application. Much greater vigilance is

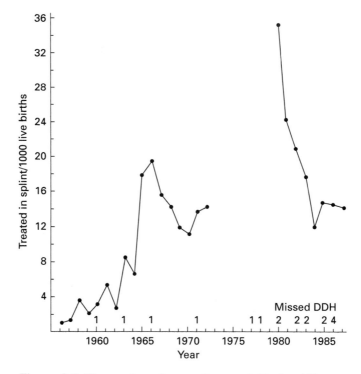

Figure 5.3 The number of cases of neonatal hip instability per 1000 births treated in a Von Rosen splint. The numbers above the line on the x axis represent the number of late cases presenting in that single year. The Barlow test was introduced into the screening programme in 1963. The authors say that the introduction of the Barlow test increases the number of cases requiring splintage without decreasing the number of late cases. (After Sanfridson *et al.*, 1991, with permission.)

needed during the first year of life if
congenital dislocation of the hip is to be
detected and treated as early as possible.
Perhaps this could be achieved if all health
professionals were more aware of the problem
and were encouraged to examine hips at every
opportunity and health authorities periodically
audited their results.

Dwyer (1987) in a personal view article was also able to call upon a large
clinical experience and very good clinical results to conclude that
improvements were necessary.

Because some of the most important organisational lessons on screening
have come from Sweden (national statistics of an accurate nature), and
because of the way they embraced the process of screening as early as
1956, a recent article indicating a fall in the efficiency of screening for DDH
must be taken very seriously indeed. Such was the article of Sanfridson *et
al.* in 1991 entitled 'Why is congenital dislocation of the hip still missed?'.
Malmo could have been described as the capital of the DDH screening
world with quite remarkable late DDH figures of 0.07 per 1000 births.
However in the 1980s this had increased to 0.6 per 1000 births, which is
a figure similar to the rest of Sweden. The authors discuss many possible
causes such as increased diagnosis (overdiagnosis), Moor's hypothesis, the
increased significance of soft tissue laxity, etc. The truth is, however, that
they are unable to explain the change but they are certain it has occurred
(Figure 5.3).

References

Catford, J.C., Bennet, G.C. and Wilkinson, J.A. (1982). Congenital hip dislocation: an
    increasing and still uncontrolled disability? *Br. Med. J. [Clin. Res.]*, **285**, 1527–1530.
Dwyer, N.St.J.P. (1987). Congenital dislocation of the hip: to screen or not to
    screen. *Arch. Dis. Child.*, **62**, 635–637.
Hadlow, V. (1988). Neonatal screening for congenital dislocation of the hip. A
    prospective 21-year survey. *J. Bone Joint Surg.*, **70B**, 740–743.
Jones, D.A. (1990). Screening for Congenital Dislocation of the Hip. MCh Thesis,
    University of Wales.
Jones, D.A. (1994). Principles of screening and congenital dislocation of the hip.
    Ann. R. Coll. Surg. Engl., **76**, 245–250.
Knox, E.G., Armstrong, E.H. and Lancashire, R.J. (1987). *Journal of Epidemiology
    and Community Health*, **41**, 283–289; 310.

Record, R.G. and Edwards, J.H. (1958). Environmental influences related to the aetiology of congenital dislocation of the hip. *Br. J. Prevt. Soc. Med.*, **12**, 8–22.
Sanfridson, J., Redlund-Johnell, I. and Udan, A. (1991). Why is congenital dislocation of the hip missed? Analysis of 96 891 infants screened in Malmo 1956–87. *Acta Orthopaedica Scandinavica*, **62**(2), 87–91.
Wilkinson, J.A. (1987). The epidemiology of congenital dislocation of the hip. *Current Orthopaedics*, **1**, 249–254.

Further reading

Jones, D.A. (1991). Neonatal hip stability and the Barlow test. A study in stillborn babies. *J. Bone Joint Surg.*, **73B**, 216–218.
Leck, I. (1986). An epidemiological assessment of neonatal screening for dislocation of the hip. *J. R. Col. Physicians Lond.*, **20**, 56–62.

6

The use of ultrasound

In this chapter an attempt will be made to put ultrasound in context as far as screening is concerned, but it has to be realised that this is a rapidly changing situation and we are very much in the most active phase of determining the place, if any, of ultrasound in the screening process for DDH. Whilst I have experience of static screening, I am not experienced in dynamic screening and it is important that this book is not considered to be a manual for those learning ultrasound.

Tip

If the reader wishes to learn the techniques of ultrasound, he or she would be well advised to seek proper hands-on training in a recognised centre. It is not something to be learned from a book and even if it was this would not be the appropriate book.

The static test

The static test works on the basis that no special manoeuvre is made but that ultrasound is simply used as a method of visualisation of the femoral head and acetabulum.

Whether or not it is as sensitive as a dynamic test remains to be seen, but the strong point in favour of the static test is that it is a true screening test, i.e. it does not require a great deal of skill that cannot easily be taught to personnel such as radiographers.

The static test can easily be carried out in the neonatal period. There are several ways in which it can be done, the method that we use is detailed below.

The baby can be examined either on a firm surface in the neonatal unit using a portable machine or in the department. The mother carries the baby into the department, keeping the baby fairly relaxed, warm and tries

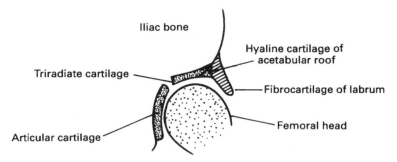

Figure 6.1 Diagram showing the ultrasound anatomy of a normal hip (Graf type 1); it should be observed in conjunction with Figure 6.2.

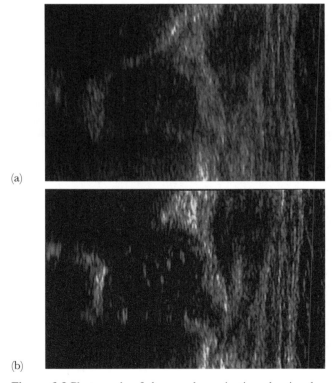

(a)

(b)

Figure 6.2 Photographs of ultrasound examinations showing the various stages of abnormality based upon the classification of Graf. For the purposes of screening, however, the Graf categories which depend upon angle measurements are not illustrated. Instead broad categories based

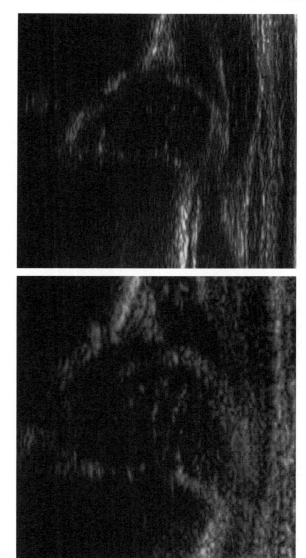

(c)

(d)

on the classification are shown. These ultrasonograms should be observed in conjunction with Figure 6.1. (a) Type 1: see Figure 6.1. (b) Type 2: the bony acetabulum is shallower and there is a larger cartilaginous component to the acetabular roof. (c) Type 3: the bony acetabulum is shallow and the labrum is displaced laterally by the femoral head. (d) Type 4: there is a large amount of displacement.

to ensure that a feed has occurred shortly before. This helps to keep the baby relaxed. The baby is then laid down on a surface which is not cold and the feet are held together by the mother or other parent in such a way that the knees are kept together and slight downward pressure is placed on the knees to put slight strain on the normal fixed flexion contracture that one finds in the neonatal hip. It must be emphasised, however, that this is not a gross degree of pressure or anything that might cause discomfort, but it simply puts a slight stress on the hips and keeps them still.

A 7.5 MHz probe is then placed over the hip in such a way as to detect the standard plane of Graf. Once the radiographer has found this plane, several hard copy ultrasonograms are taken. The same is then done on the opposite hip. This procedure takes approximately 1 minute per hip.

The radiographer can be trained to read these ultrasonograms using the classification of Graf but without drawing any lines and using the method of global visual analysis described by Zeigler (this really means that one is eye-balling the ultrasonogram and putting the result into approximate groupings). For this test to be ideal as a screening test, the whole procedure and the report should be carried out by a radiographer. In Swansea we are currently going over to this method after a period of investigation of the reliability of the radiographers in doing these reports. At present, all abnormal reports are verified by the radiologist and a system has been instituted whereby the radiographer alerts the clinical staff if there is any evidence of anything other than a type 1 or normal hip.

The use of the Graf classification for the purposes of screening is demonstrated in Figures 6.1 and 6.2.

The dynamic test

The dynamic test as described by Graf (Graf, 1984) is as follows. A real time ultrasound instrument is required and

> the behaviour of the femoral head in the
> immature acetabulum gives the examiner
> important information with regard to further
> therapy thus, when the joint is examined
> under pressure an attempt is made to push
> the femoral head posteriorly or superiorly out
> of the acetabulum. The examiner notes
> whether this produces only an elastic deflexion
> of the labrum, or whether a marked
> displacement of the femoral head is elicited.

He then goes on to describe two abnormalities.

1. Elastic deflexion

Graf states that even in fully mature hips there might be slight upward elastic deflexion of the labrum during movement of the proximal femur but a true dislocation is not possible.

2. Sonographic instability sign

When the contour of the bony acetabular roof is severely deficient but with a good, wide overhang of cartilage rim, it is usual to be able to show some degree of sonographic instability. When upward pressure is applied to the femur during the examination, the head of the femur can be observed to slip out of the primary acetabular roof and displace the wide cartilaginous roof posteriorly or superiorly. When the pressure is released, the head slips back to its original position. Sonographic instability does not necessarily correlate with clinical instability and is far more sensitive. It also gives a visual output on the screen, whereas clinical interpretation depends upon the tactile ability of the examiner. It was Graf's opinion in 1994 that an ultrasound stability test should be performed on all hips that are documented to be at least type 2 in the Graf grades of abnormality.

The method which has found more generalised acceptance is that of Harcke et al. (1984). The method is well described, together with the classification of the result, in a paper by Marks et al. (1994).

The screening in their case was carried out by senior radiographers using a 7.5 MHz short focus linear ray transducer. Two images of each hip were made and recorded by thermal image printing. The baby is supine and the pelvis flat. The coronal/flexion view is taken with the hip and knee flexed to 90 degrees and the transducer aligned at 90 degrees to the femur.

The transverse/neutral view is obtained with the hip and knee extended and the transducer rotated through 90 degrees, i.e. perpendicular to the long axis of the body. No form of provocation test was carried out and no clinical examination made by the radiographer. The grading used was that described by Terjesen et al. (1989).

Who and when?

With ultrasound screening, the first screening examination is best done in the immediate neonatal period, because it is designed to find out two things: (i) whether the acetabulum is mature and normal and (ii) whether there is any evidence of instability. The implication is that if, at that stage, there is no abnormality of the hip, either structural or functional, then those babies can be safely discharged and further examinations are only applied to babies who have an initial abnormality.

If this is so, then clearly the answer is that the examination ought to be done before the baby is discharged from hospital and, in order to satisfy the needs of a screening test, it should be done not by senior medical personnel but by radiographers.

The ultrasound test should be carried out in the immediate neonatal period soon after birth and before the child leaves hospital. At present, the test may be carried out by professionals in one or more of four specialities: (i) radiographers; (ii) radiologists; (iii) orthopaedic surgeons, and (iv) paediatricians.

The involvement of senior medical personnel is of course quite legitimate when the test is in its period of development but once that development has occurred it would be an inappropriate use of resources for a senior member of the medical staff to be carrying out routine screening examinations using ultrasound. That is not to say that it would not be quite reasonable and proper for medical staff to be involved in the further assessment of abnormal hips.

The question as to who does the test, is very important and if it is a screening test it should be done by the lowest grade of personnel who can be trained to competently carry out that test. This should be a qualified radiographer and clearly for practical reasons within any department, it would mean that several radiographers must be trained to carry it out and to do it at regular intervals.

Early results of ultrasound screening

At the outset, it has to be stated that no firm conclusion can be drawn at this stage as to whether ultrasound is going to be a valuable adjunct to examination in screening for DDH.

The signals are ambivalent and different studies have given different degrees of hope in this respect. Part of the problem has been that because of the resource implications ultrasound tests have been applied only in the at-risk group and results have been further confused by the use of ultrasound of a static nature and also ultrasound of a dynamic nature, although the majority of workers in this field have now gone on to dynamic testing as a routine. When the results of screening are recorded and described in research papers, it is extremely important that the figure which is given relates to the population of births, and not simply a population which happens to be studied.

The present state of ultrasound in relationship to DDH screening is well summarised in an editorial by Catterall (1994). Ultrasound examination was first introduced in the early 1980s (Graf, 1984), and enthusiasts regarded this as being 'the solution'. The advantage of ultrasound over radiology was, firstly, that there was no irradiation but, more importantly, it was able to visualise cartilaginous structures more directly. Adding ultrasound imaging to clinical examination at birth increases the number of abnormal hips detected, but most of these abnormalities would have got better in any event without treatment and one of the criticisms of ultrasound is that it may detect more abnormalities of this sort without increasing the diagnosis of the cases which are going to develop into late DDH. (Screening for scoliosis fell out of favour for this reason.)

Some papers have looked at every birth rather than simply births selected on the basis of risk factors; e.g. in Marks *et al.* (1994), 6% of infants had abnormal scans but 90% of these had become normal by the age of 9 weeks, resulting in a figure of 0.85 per 1000 persisting ultrasound abnormalities.

The current evidence is that ultrasound examination, whether it involves the whole population or at-risk groups, does not give better results on a population basis than the results of careful clinical examination using radiography at 3–4 months when indicated. Catterall concluded:

> at present the cornerstone of diagnosis must
> be the clinical examination of all infants by
> experts on at least two occasions in the first 3
> months of life. Ultrasound examination may
> be justifiable for the at risk population to
> which may be added infants born by
> Caesarean Section and those treated in special
> care units.

Catterall concludes that an ultrasound examination should demonstrate both dysplasia and instability and seems to be recommending the classification of Terjesen *et al.* (1989). A summary of the results of various methods of population screening is contained in Table 6.1.

Table 6.1 Results of various methods of screening

Paper	Screening method	Late DDH rate per 1000 births	Birth cohort
Hadlow, 1988	Clinical examination	0.09	20 000
Boeree and Clarke, 1994	Dynamic ultrasound	0.22	26 952
Fiddian and Gardner, 1994	Clinical examination by physiotherapists	0.3	42 241
Lewis Jones and Powell, 1995	Static ultrasound	0.33	17 793
Clark et al., 1989	Dynamic ultrasound	0.68	4617
McKenzie, 1972	Clinical examination	1.12	76 675

Taken from Lewis, C., Jones, D. A. and Powell, N. (personal communication).

References

Boeree, N.R. and Clarke, N.M. (1994). Ultrasound imaging and secondary screening for congenital dislocation of the hip. *J. Bone Joint Surg.*, **76B**, 525–533.

Catterall, A. (1994). The early diagnosis of congenital dislocation of the hip. *J. Bone Joint Surg.*, **76B**, 515–516.

Clarke, N.M., Clegg, J. and Al-Chalabi, A.N. (1989). Ultrasound screening of hips at risk for CDH. Failure to reduce the incidence of late cases. *J. Bone Joint Surg.*, **71B**, 9–12.

Fiddian, N.J. and Gardiner, J.C. (1994). Screening for congenital dislocation of the hip by physiotherapists. Results of a ten-year study. *J. Bone Joint Surg.*, **76B**, 458–459.

Graf, R. (1984). Classification of hip joint dysplasia by means of sonography. *Archives of Orthopaedic and Trauma Surgery*, **102**, 248–255.

Graf, R. (1984) The ultrasound examination of the hip. In *Congenital Dysplasia and Dislocation of the Hip* (D. Tönnis, ed.) Berlin: Springer Verlag, 172–229.

Graf, R. (1984). Fundamentals of sonographic diagnosis of infant hip dysplasia. *J. Pediatr. Orthop.*, **4**, 735–740.

Harcke, H.T., Clark, N.M., Lee, M.S., Borns, P.F. and MacEwen, G.D. (1984). Examination of the infant hip with real time ultrasonography. *J. Ultrasound Med.*, **4**, 131–137.

Marks, D.S., Clegg, J. and Al-Chalabi, A.N. (1994). Routine ultrasound screening for neonatal hip instability. Can it abolish late-presenting congenital dislocation of the hip? *J. Bone Joint Surg.*, **76B**, 534–538.

McKenzie, I.G. (1972). Congenital dislocation of the hip: the development of a regional service. *J. Bone Joint Surg.*, **54B**, 18–39.

Terjesen ,T, Bredland, T. and Berg, V. (1989). Ultrasound for hip assessment in the newborn. *J. Bone Joint Surg.*, **71**, 767–773.

Further reading

Clarke, N.M.P. (1992). Diagnosing congenital dislocation of the hip – a large trial of ultrasonography might help. *Br. Med. J.*, **305**, 435.

Harcke, H.T. (1992). Imaging in congenital dislocation and dysplasia of the hip. [Review]. *Clin. Orthop. Rel. Res.*, 22–28.

Jones, D.A. and Powell, N. (1990). Ultrasound and neonatal hip screening. A prospective study of 'high risk' babies. *J. Bone Joint Surg.*, **72**, 457–459.

Knox, E.G., Armstrong, E.H. and Lancashire, R.J. (1987). Effectiveness of screening for congenital dislocation of the hip. *J. Epidemiol. Community Health*, **41**, 283–289.

Zieger, M., Hilpert, S. and Schulz, R.D. (1986). Ultrasound of the infant hip. Part 2. Validity of the method. *Pediatr. Radiol.*, **16**, 488–492.

7

Ethical and legal considerations

There are of course both ethical and legal implications in screening.

Ethical implications

It was pointed out many years ago by Cochrane that screening is very different from all other forms of medical intervention. Screening is done on the basis that its outcome is inevitably good. Generally, no specific consent is obtained, there is a general presumption that the process is in the interests of the child being examined and, providing the test is harmless and the subsequent treatment is harmless, there can be no great ethical objection to this taking place.

However, the question must be asked whether, if an examination is designed with the best possible motives in mind, one should automatically assume consent in order to do this examination.

Considerable reservations must be present for an adult. When he/she goes to a doctor with a complaint this naturally implies consent to examination and that he/she is fully in agreement with that examination, i.e. he/she does not have to sign a consent form to say he/she is going to be examined, provided no invasive techniques are used.

The parent would be the legal guardian of the baby and, therefore, it is important to ask the parent whether they agree to this examination being carried out. This is particularly important if there is any risk, however small, that the examination may be harmful. It is also particularly true if there is no overwhelming evidence that the examination is likely to detect the condition which is being looked for, i.e. it is very much less ethically acceptable if the test is of low sensitivity. How does one get around these difficult problems? One way, and in my opinion a very good way and a method that we have instituted in Swansea, is to give parents of all neonates an information sheet at the time of birth. The information sheet points out the nature of screening for DDH, reminding the parents of the risk factors and, in particular, reminding them that the clinical

SWANSEA NHS TRUST - SINGLETON HOSPITAL
SCREENING FOR CONGENITAL DISLOCATION OF THE HIP
INFORMATION LEAFLET
FOR PARENTS OF NEWBORN BABIES

Abnormality of the hip occurs in about 15 children per thousand born. Most of these do not matter and will self-correct, but some of them (2 per thousand) lead to dislocation of the hip.

In this hospital we have a special system called **SCREENING** which attempts to detect and therefore prevent dislocation of the hip and its consequences.

If your baby has any of the following risk factors an **ULTRASOUND SCAN** will be arranged:

[1]	Family history of dislocation of the hip	)
		)
[2]	Breech position (not simply breech birth)	)
		)
[3]	Caesarean section (for breech)	)
		)
[4]	Postural foot deformities	) 10%
		) births
[5]	Oligohydramnios (dry birth)	)
		)
[6]	Clicking hips	)
		)
[7]	Any concern by the paediatricians on examining the hips	)

Even if the hips are found to be normal on examination, it is still important that the hips are examined by your GP at the subsequent routine examinations during the first year of life.

Even with the excellent facilities we have available, the screening programme is not 100% accurate. It is therefore most important that the hips are examined after you leave hospital by your own GP or Clinical Medical Officer at the 6 weeks and 7/8 months routine examination.

You may rest assured that in this area our record is extremely good, but it is felt that every parent should have access to the information in this handout so that they can understand what the doctors are doing when they are examining babies hips.

Directorate of	Directorate of
Child Health	Paediatric Orthopaedics

Figure 7.1 Example of an information leaflet for screening for DDH in the newborn.

examination in itself is not 100% effective in eliminating the develop-mental dysplasia of the hip and making it very clear that further examinations would be necessary during the early months of life (Figure 7.1).

If the parents have such an information leaflet then it is not unreasonable to assume consent if they have read that before the examination is carried out. The examiner however must be prepared to answer the following questions:

1. Is the test harmful? The answer to this is that it is probably not harmful providing it is not done repeatedly or forcefully and therefore it is implicit in this statement that the examiner has been trained to do the examination.
2. Does the test always find the condition? The answer to this question is clearly 'no' and this must be followed by an explanation that the screening process is a series of examinations or assessments.
3. Does my baby require an ultrasound scan? The answer to this question does depend to some extent on the facilities available but it is an opportunity to indicate and remind the parent of the risk factors which might put the baby into a group where most would agree an ultrasound scan is indicated.

In the unlikely event that a parent does not wish the child's hips to be examined on the basis of screening then, in my opinion, this request should be complied with; however, gentle persuasion should again be tried but if the parent does not want this examination then one would have to say that on the balance of probabilities, based upon our present results, one could not make out a very strong case for overpersuading them to take part. *Perhaps what is more important under these circumstances is to point out how important it is for a simple examination measuring the degree of abduction to be carried out at the 8-week stage.*

Legal considerations and the concept of blame

There was undoubtedly a period in the history of screening where it was strongly believed by the protagonists of screening that it was always possible to detect any tendency to DDH at the neonatal examination. Such enthusiasts found it difficult to believe that it is possible for the condition to develop insidiously over the early months of life, but there is now good clinical and ultrasonic proof that the latter can occur.

It is not surprising therefore that young doctors in particular felt very vulnerable in the performance of the tests to detect neonatal hip instability and this also acted as a very strong deterrent for other health professionals to get closely involved in an area which could prove to have unpleasant legal implications for those who 'missed' positive cases. It is difficult to know precisely what effect this had and how it influenced the way in which screening developed. There are three areas which merit discussion:

(a) Failure to diagnose the condition.
(b) Failure to fully document the examination.
(c) The legal status of clinical guidelines.

Failure to diagnose in the neonatal period

This is well illustrated by the following legal case.

The case of H. N. T

The principles here are well illustrated by a case which appeared before the Supreme Court of Alabama published on 19 June 1992. Dr D was sued by the parents of H. N. T because he had failed to diagnose a congenital hip dislocation. The jury returned a verdict in favour of Dr D but the plaintiffs appealed asking for a new trial. That trial was granted but Dr D appealed and it is the subject of this appeal in which the evidence is reviewed. The question at issue was whether Dr D in failing to diagnose the congenital dislocation of the hip deviated from a medically accepted standard of care at the time. H. was 4 months old when first seen by Dr D. Several other doctors had previously examined H. and Dr D had examined her several times in a 14-month period. Eight of the nine visits were for specific illnesses which were unrelated to her hips. H. went to see another paediatrician, Dr K, who examined H. and found a dislocated hip. H. was then referred to Dr E, a paediatric orthopaedist, who undertook surgery to correct the problem.

The expert evidence was as follows: Dr G for the plaintiffs said that Dr D should have diagnosed the condition and testified that the earlier the diagnosis the better the outcome. Dr G indicated that the diagnosis was made more easily in the first 28 days of life.

The expert for the plaintiffs, Dr B, testified that in Dr D's report he could find no record of a thorough examination of H.'s musculoskeletal system and failure to do such an examination was a deviation from the accepted standard of care. Dr R presented expert testimony on behalf of Dr D and stated that there was a different type of examination given to a sick baby than the type given to a well baby and this statement was agreed by all the medical experts. Dr E, the paediatric orthopaedist, testified that

H.'s dislocated hip had been present since birth and that Dr D's failure to diagnose the dislocated hip did not cause any additional injury.

The conclusion was that it was fairly easily perceivable from the record that the jury's verdict for Dr D was supported by sufficient evidence. Dr R testified that Dr D met the appropriate standard of care. It was also stated that when a child is ill it is not necessary for the doctor to examine the hips on every visit. Dr R testified that it is possible to do an adequate examination and still not detect a dislocated hip and they also took account of Dr G's testimony that a dislocated hip is easier to detect in the first 28 days of life.

It is thought that the commonest cause of litigation brought against paediatricians in the USA is failure to diagnose DDH. They go on to point out that in Europe the system of fault liability implicates an obligation of ability and means. *Failure to diagnose or misdiagnosis is not a fault in itself as long as a complete history, careful physical examination and adequate and appropriate complimentary examinations have been performed by an adequately trained physician.*

Comment

If congenital hip dislocation is recognised and treated early, most of the affected children will develop functionally and radiologically normal hips, but the caveat is added that this is not always the case and early treatment is not always successful or without complication and therefore damages due to late onset of the treatment are difficult to assess.

The above reported case represents my understanding of the present view that Courts may take in terms of what is and what is not proper in terms of DDH practice:

1. It has to be accepted that it is not always possible to diagnose the condition clinically at birth and there is good evidence to indicate that this is so.
2. Even if diagnosis is made it does not always result well and complications can still occur.

There are certain points, however, that any screener must bear in mind and can be called to account, and these are:

1. That an adequate history was taken and that risk factors were noted.
2. That a proper examination was carried out.
3. That the results of that proper examination were documented and that later complementary examinations are performed.
4. The screeners must satisfy themselves that they fall within the definition of adequately and appropriate trained personnel.

As far as I can see, there are several things in this set of circumstances which are open to interpretation. Firstly, what is an appropriate examination and, secondly, what is an appropriately trained person.

An appropriate examination would consist of carrying out one of the tests of instability at birth and recording very carefully all the features such as leg length, extra skin creases, whether the hip clicks or not, and whether there is any indication of instability. The way things are at the moment the Barlow test and the Ortolani test are really described as one but I would have thought it would have been essential to have done at least one of these tests, and probably both, in the neonatal period. However, as time passes later screening examinations might call for less stringent examination in this sense but a more stringent examination in terms of measurement of the degree of abduction.

What is an appropriately qualified person? This is difficult to say; at the present time paediatric senior house officers are the usual examiners and to some extent in this country they must be regarded as the benchmark. Each one has to demonstrate that he/she has had adequate training.

If other examiners such as health visitors, midwives and physiotherapists, carry out the test, then it is important they have and can be shown to have had, the appropriate training. This might prove difficult in the UK, as in 50% of health authorities no designated officer has been identified but, generally, most people working locally in an area will understand which physician or surgeon has an interest in this particular area.

It would appear that the actual professional group of such a person is not relevant, but what is more relevant is that they are persons who have been specifically instructed and trained in this area and there is increasing evidence that they would.

The legal case described a very interesting case and illustrates many principles, perhaps the most important of which is that whenever an examination is done, whoever does it, then an adequate record of that examination is essential in legal terms (and in my opinion also in medical terms).

The courts therefore seem to accept the following principles when given to them in medical evidence:

1. That an adequate examination may still not detect a dislocated hip in the early months of life.
2. That it is easier to detect a dislocated hip in the first 28 days than afterwards (this point could be contested, but what the medical experts are saying is clear – that the dislocatability becomes a less good physical

sign with the passage of time. I think the possibility that the tightness of the adductors would take over and make the diagnosis more easy to make was overlooked.)

Failure to fully document the examination

This is well illustrated by the following legal case.

The case of P. R

This case was heard at the Appelate Court of Illinois, First District, Fifth Division, on 14 September 1990. The mother alleged that Dr S was negligent in failing to diagnose and treat P.'s bilateral congenital hip dislocation. The case was complicated somewhat by the presence of the child in the neonatal intensive care unit, but Dr S examined the child within 12 hours of birth when there were clear medical problems. At no time during this admission to the intensive care unit did Dr S note anything in P.'s medical chart relating to his hips or discuss the hips with mother. The boy's mother testified that when P. was 1 month old she noticed that his right foot turned outwards. The condition did not change and she had P. examined by an orthopaedic specialist at about 6 months of age when the diagnosis of congenital dislocated hips was made and treatment began. In evidence, Dr S described in detail her normal examination of the hips, mentioning both the Ortolani test and the Barlow test. She admitted in evidence that early diagnosis was helpful in obtaining an excellent outcome. Dr S estimated that 1–5% of babies might not have an abnormality diagnosable at birth and later present with a congenital dislocation. She indicated that the Barlow test was not 100% sensitive. The medical records, however, showed no specific entry regarding the hips. She indicated she only records positive findings and not negative findings but said she could recall doing a complete and thorough physical examination. The expert witness called by the plaintiff said that he had no opinion which was critical of Dr S and had no opinion at all with regard to the care and treatment of P. by the hospital.

In this case the action against Dr S failed, largely because of lack of expert testimony to indicate any criticism of her behaviour. Nevertheless, it was clear in the proceedings that it would have been much better if she had made an accurate record of exactly what examination she carried out and she may be regarded as fortunate that medical evidence was not produced which would have been critical of this fact.

Comment

It would be surprising if any court would find a doctor, or other health professional, negligent for failing to diagnose a dislocatable hip at birth in a patient who later presents with a so-called 'missed' DDH.

Although the legal precedent in cases of DDH is very limited and largely confined to the American literature, there are undoubtedly lessons to be learned and these are:

1. The documentation must always be good and complete for every child.
2. Any hint of an abnormality should be considered reason to proceed to an ultrasound scan.
3. The parents should always be informed that any one examination at any point in time does not constitute a guarantee that the condition of DDH will not show itself later and therefore should be encouraged to keep appointments for subsequent examinations.

The legal status of clinical guidelines

If the screening policy in any individual area is well defined then it is very difficult for this to occur efficiently without producing clinical guidelines. For example, such guidelines might indicate precisely who should do the screening, when and how it should be recorded, etc. A further set of guidelines would indicate precisely what action should be taken, depending on the clinical findings, and what further action should be taken in terms of secondary screening when primary screening does not yield a positive result.

The question arises as to what legal liability there is on the professionals carrying out this work if they do not adhere to the guidelines. Indeed the question has to be asked if there is any degree of safety to healthcare workers if they stick within the guidelines. As stated earlier, the standard of clinical care required by law is generally that judged reasonable and proper by a body of responsible doctors as ascertained in court from expert testimony. A similar principle would apply to other healthcare workers, but there is an added complication in screening, and that is to what extent the responsibility is delegated by whom and to whom. For example, is it the health authority that decides whether or not neonatal screening is done by a paediatric doctor or by a paediatric physiotherapist for example. Or is it the case that the consultant paediatrician delegates this task to a physiotherapist, or indeed, under the terms of the 1986 report, would it not be the designated officer who decides who should do what and when.

The status of guidelines is that they are classed as hearsay evidence, so in British courts no decision is made as to what is reasonable and proper care simply by referring to them. In a recent leading article in the *British Medical Journal*, Brian Hurwitz (1995) stated:

> However impressive the organisation that
> sponsored the guidelines, or its process for
> developing them, the fact that a protocol
> exists for a particular condition does not mean
> that what it proposes is true. Nor does it
> guarantee that the protocol accurately
> represents customary practice.

He quotes two important legal cases where British judges have not automatically equated established guidelines with reasonable and proper medical practice (*Earley* v. *Newham Health Authority* 1994; *Loveday* v. *Renton and Welcome Foundation Limited* (QBD) 1990).

In legal terms the following questions may be asked of any set of guidelines:

1. How was it developed and adopted?
2. What is the mandatory force of its recommendations?
3. Are there any known exceptions to its application?
4. Is there any school of medical thought which rejects it and adopts a different approach?

Courts might naturally like the idea of guidelines because it is fairly easy to decide whether or not they were complied with. However, courts have shown that whilst they like them they also like to retain the power to overrule them. There is no evidence that the presence of guidelines fuels litigation, which was one of the worries in the American system, and a recent survey showed that in American malpractice cases clinical guidelines played a relevant and pivotal role in the proof of negligence in about 6.6% of cases (Hymans *et al.*, 1995).

The general conclusion appears to be that, on the whole, guidelines are a good thing. They are more protective of the health professional involved in screening than they are a threat to him or her. The current view of Kennedy is that the role of protocols and guidelines will become more and more significant in determining whether a doctor has violated the law.

In summary, therefore, it would appear that if clinical guidelines for

DDH screening help and they are drawn up properly, and considered properly, then they are not likely to in any way make the screeners more liable to litigation. It would appear that the reverse is the case, that it would give the screeners some degree of protection provided they complied with the guidelines, but may possibly make them more vulnerable to litigation if they do not comply with the guidelines.

The following situation is one which might cause some concern. Let us say a screener worked in a health authority that did not have any particular guidelines on screening and did not have available ultrasound. At present there are probably many such authorities and their incidence of undetected DDH will be much higher than authorities where a proper well controlled screening programme has been instituted with the use of ultrasound.

Let us take a high risk case such as a baby born by breech birth having been in a breech position. This is known to be a high risk case and in health authority (A) such a case would be treated very much like any other case, except that there might be more clinical alertness to the possibility of an abnormality. If an abnormality remained undetected, providing the examinations were all carried out and documented properly, it is unlikely that there would be any basis for litigation.

In health authority (B) however, where the guidelines are clear that such a baby would be referred for a neonatal ultrasound scan, the question arises as to whether the screener is negligent by not referring such a person for an ultrasound scan.

I know in my own unit there have been many cases where for reasons of business etc., the paediatric senior house officers have failed to elicit family histories of neonatal hip problems and scans have gone undone which otherwise would have been done. It is unclear whether this particular situation would lead to vulnerability to legal action and as far as I am aware such cases are untested in law at the present time.

References

Cochrane, A.L. (1989). Effectiveness and efficiency. Random reflections on health sevices. *Brit. Med. J.*

Cochrane, A.L. and Holland, W.W. (1971). Validation of screening procedures. *Br. Med. Bull.*, **27**, 3–8.

Earley v. *Newham Health Authority* (1994). 5 Medical Law Reports, 215–217.

Hurwitz, B. (1995). Clinical guidelines and the law. *Br. Med. J.*, **311**, 1517–1518.

Hymans, A.L., Brandenburgh, J.A., Lipsitz, S.R., Shapiro, D.W. and Brennan,

T.A. (1995). Practice guidelines and malpractice litigation: a two way street. *Ann. Intern. Med.*, **122**, 450–455.

Kennedy, I. (1993). Medicine in society now and in the future. In *Eighty-five not out. Essays to Honour Sir George Godfer* (S. Lock, ed.) London: King Edward's Hospital Fund for London, 69–75.

Loveday v. *Renton and Welcome Foundation Limited (QBD)* (1990). 1 Med LR, 117–204.

8

Cost and psychology

Like most treatments or diagnostic tests, there is a negative side to screening as well as the more obvious positive side. In a modern context almost everything has to be justified on the basis of cost. There have been attempts to analyse the cost of the whole screening process and then to set against it the costs of carrying out the operations which would have been required had screening not been carried out. This is a difficult matter, however. Firstly, it is virtually impossible to know precisely what the costs of clinics that would be occurring in any event really are and what extra costs there are in carrying out certain extra tests. Secondly, there is the problem of knowing in population terms whether there are true savings in the number of late cases in the country as a whole and whether detecting them earlier really saves money. It is probably possible to manipulate the figures in such a way to give whichever answer you wish, but of the studies that have been carried out the majority seem to indicate that the process of screening is about cost neutral, i.e. it is not a procedure that should be carried out with the prime aim of saving money. This of course very much fits in with the ethical view that the main purpose of screening for a condition such as DDH is that if the condition can be detected earlier it should be, and if early treatment is better than late treatment then it is early treatment we should be aiming at. These values are much more to do with our tradition of caring professions than they are with the more modern accountant-like attitude which seems to be prevailing.

Of course there is a psychological benefit for parents knowing that an attempt is being made to find out whether their child has a problem. However, there is a psychological cost of the anxiety created in the family of every false positive case discovered on screening, i.e. these are cases which are not really abnormal at all but because of the insensitivity of the tests there is a suspicion expressed as to whether the hip is normal or abnormal and until this suspicion is totally clarified the parents and others in the family are subjected to a psychological adverse experience. If the number of false positives is high, then the total damage done could be quite considerable. It may also be argued that there is a considerable psychological blow dealt to those parents who are reassured that their babies' hips are normal only to find out later that they are not normal. These of course are the false negatives.

Psychological costs of screening

This subject has been excellently reviewed by Marteau. She points out that a positive result in any screening test is invariably received with negative feelings. In the case of a false positive result, i.e. the case where in subsequent examinations and tests the baby is found not to have the disease, it might be expected that this discovery would be a source of relief. However, there have been studies in subjects other than DDH which indicate that once the seeds of doubt have been sown the parents find them difficult to remove and they may be a long-term source of insecurity. This was certainly found to be true for the discovery of heart murmurs on routine examination.

The negative result of the screening examination can also have an undesirable effect. For example, it could be interpreted by the parents that the baby is being given a complete bill of health for the indefinite future and there is some evidence that this may act as a reason to reinforce an unhealthy lifestyle. There has been very little research done on the importance of counselling before screening and many have concluded that, unless the emotional and behavioural consequences of screening programmes are properly monitored, we will remain uncertain of their overall value.

The actual psychological effects are usually revealed in the form of high levels of anxiety and this can be reflected by an increase in consultation rates, etc. For some patients even being told of the possibility of an abnormality can be distressing. There is virtually no research on the effects of the false negative result and the false positive result and yet these are really quite well defined situations.

Various means have been suggested to reduce the psychological effects and these are largely to do with counselling and information and other time consuming methods. It is all to do with providing information in various forms and making sure that the participants understand this information. It is suggested that the following information should be given to the patient or the parents before a screening test is carried out:

1. The condition being screened for.
2. The test procedure.
3. When and how the results are available.

4. The likelihood of a positive result.
5. The meaning of both negative and positive results.
6. Action for those with a positive result.

The method by which the results are given can also be extremely important. It is generally assumed, and certainly practice, for good results to be given at a less senior level than bad results. The actual delivery of the result could be by telephone, by post, during a pre-arranged appointment or possibly even an unscheduled home visit, depending upon the particular disease being screened for. With DDH it is usually an instant result but sometimes in some circumstances a result from say an ultrasound scan or an X-ray may involve some delay. There are therefore important implications for staff training.

Marteau suggests the following criteria should be adhered to, bearing in mind psychological costs, in any screening programme:

1. Prepare a written protocol covering all aspects of screening.
2. Train staff.
3. Issue motivating – not threatening – invitations and reminders.
4. Give information orally and in writing before the test.
5. Inform all patients of their test results.
6. Follow up all patients with positive results.
7. Evaluate both epidemiological and psychological outcomes of the programme.

There is one other psychological matter, however, which must be considered. It has been pointed out in Chapter 7, relating to ethics – that screening differs very much from other forms of medical intervention in that it is initiated by the profession. If, having initiated such a procedure and found a problem and then, as a result of finding that problem, treatment is begun which itself has complications which in turn result in a condition which might be worse than the untreated disease, this is something which has great ethical and psychological consequences. Unfortunately this is possible in DDH and the disease complication is avascular necrosis of the femoral head. Fortunately this is not a common complication of early splintage but it can occur, to some extent, with nearly all splints.

Financial costs of screening

Leck, in his assessment of this subject, quotes the figures from British Columbia in 1981/1982 and applied the method to the Bristol statistics published by Dunn *et al.* (1985) and concluded that the ratio of the costs with screening to costs without screening is approximately 0.97 to 1, indicating a marginal benefit for screening.

In a detailed analysis in British Columbia, Treadwell (1990) indicated that for every 1000 infants born there was an economic benefit of screening of over 15 000 Canadian dollars but this does depend on having a very low false negative rate as shown in Figure 1.5.

In discussing financial costs and psychological costs an assumption is made, which is a reasonable assumption, that, generally, the results of treatment are good.

In conclusion, therefore, it would appear that there are marginal cost benefits for screening when the screening programme is shown to be fairly successful. There are fairly major psychological costs and there has been very little research on this, although it is an area where further research would be most welcome.

References

Treadwell, S.J. (1990). Economic evaluation of neonatal screening for congenital dislocation of the hip. *J. Pediatr. Orthop.*, **10**, 326–330.

Further reading

Cairns, J. (1995). The costs of prevention. *Br. Med. J.*, **311**, 1520.

Dunn, P.M., Evans, R.E., Thearle, M.J. *et al.* (1985). Congenital dislocation of the hip: early and late diagnosis and management compared. *Archives of Disease in Childhood*, **60**(5), 407–414.

Catford, J.C., Bennett, G.C. and Wilkinson, J.A. (1982). Congenital dislocation of the hip: an increasing and still uncontrolled disability. *Br. Med. J.*, **285**, 1527–1530.

Edwards, P.J. and Hall, D.M.B. (1992). Screening, ethics and the law. *Br. Med. J.*, **305**, 267–268.

Leck, I. (1986). An epidemiological assessment of neonatal screening for dislocation of the hip. *J. R. Coll. Physicians Lond.*, **20**, 56–62.

Marteau, T.M. (1989). Psychological costs of screening. Editorial. *Br. Med. J.*, **299**, 527.

Marteau, T.M. (1990). Reducing the psychological cost. Editorial. *Br. Med. J.*, **301**, 26–28.

Sackett, D. and Holland, W.W. (1975). Controversy in the detection of disease. *Lancet*, **ii**, 357–359.

9

Organisation documentation and computerisation

One of the main recommendations of the 1986 report of the Standing Medical Advisory Committee and the Standing Nursing and Midwifery Advisory Committee for the Secretaries of State for Social Services and for Wales, in a booklet entitled 'Screening for the Detection of Congenital Dislocation of the Hip', was that in each district, as defined by a District Health Authority, there should be a clear policy outlining who is responsible for undertaking the examination for DDH at the ages outlined and for passing the results or notification that the examination has not been done to the GP and the community midwife or health visitor. The ages outlined were: (i) within 24 hours of birth; (ii) at the time of discharge from hospital; (iii) at 6 weeks; (iv) between 6 and 9 months; (v) between 15 and 21 months.

The report went on to recommend that a designated officer within each district should keep the whole screening programme under review and record and evaluate the incidence of cases detected late. Such information should be made available to the health professionals concerned.

From further work (Jones *et al.*, 1991) it is known that 50% of health authorities had not heeded that recommendation some 2 years after the publication of the report. Therefore there is a real problem with the organisation of screening programmes in the UK. What should be recorded?

At the neonatal examination within 24 hours of birth:

1. Is there a family history?
2. Was the baby at any time in the breech position?
3. On the examination, was the Roser–Le Damaney–Ortolani–Barlow test normal or abnormal?
4. Were any clicks or clunks elicited?
5. Was there any sign of fetal moulding either in the feet or the head or the spine?
6. Was there full abduction of the hips?
7. Were the skin creases symmetrical in the thighs and in the perianal region?

At the 6–8 month examination the questions which must be asked are:

1. Is there any leg length discrepancy?
2. Is there any skin crease asymmetry?
3. Is there any thigh shortening or telescoping?
4. Is there any evidence of instability of the hip?
5. What is the range of abduction? (a) 0–60 degrees; (b) 60–80 degrees; (c) >80 degrees?
6. Is there any difference between the left and right sides?

The value of asking questions of this sort is that they can easily be contained in a proforma or stamped onto the parent-held child record and are ideal for computerisation. Computers are at their best in dealing with simple yes/no answers or answers that result in a figure, e.g. degrees of abduction. Even in this case it is better to offer a range, e.g. What is the range of hip abduction: (a) <60 degrees; (b) 60–80 degrees; (c) >80 degrees? This option should be noted separately for the right and left hip. A computer program could then easily pick out certain patterns, e.g. restricted abduction on one side.

Tip

If you are organising a screening programme and you wish to try to get some form of computerised audit of the process, you will find the following difficulties:
1. Community health services, GPs and hospitals have computer systems which do not communicate.
2. The 'returns' filled in for community health are often lacking in space and you will be told 'there is no room' and you may be offered one line only!
3. It is almost impossible to get all the information you need together in one place at one time.

A possible proforma which would be suitable for scanning into a computer is shown in Figure 9.1.

The organisation of the neonatal examinations will inevitably differ from place to place. The recommendation is that these babies are all examined together in a side ward where the staff are aware of the need for the baby to be fully relaxed on a flat surface, etc., and the examiner can then comfortably sit down, elicit all the historical data and carry out the examination. This is greatly to be preferred to the method of going around the wards and examining the babies in a bedside situation where

Risk factor(s) present	Yes	No

Family history	
Clicking hip	
Breech position *in utero*	
Postural deformity	
Joint hyperlaxity	
Other	

Skin creases	Symmetrical	Non-symmetrical
Thigh		
Buttocks		

Asymmetrical inguinal creases

Ando and Goto grade	Right	Left
A		
B		
C		
D		

Abduction range	*Right*	*Left*
60		
60–80		
>80		

Feature	*Normal*	*Abnormal*
Ortolani		
Barlow		
Telescoping		
Leg length		

Range	Right	Left
<60		
B60–80		
C >80		

Figure 9.1 DDH screening programme – data collection at 8 weeks.

there is a great temptation to examine the baby in the cot rather than on a flat surface.

As a result of this examination, in many areas all babies with risk factors or any suspicion of abnormality on clinical examination will then be referred for an ultrasound scan. The result of this examination must be put in the clinical record, transcribed into the parent-held record and sent on a computer friendly form to some central source such as the district community health computer so that the information is centralised.

At the present time there is no special facility within the child health record for hip screening, but a strong case could be made out for a separate page being devoted to this subject. Also at the present time the computer input forms do not allow a great deal of information about the hip examination to be recorded, but it is a small matter for this to be put right and there is a strong case for doing so.

Documentation

The clinical neonatal record is obviously the documentation in which the hand-written result of the screening examination will be recorded. Unfortunately, all too often it is the only place where it is recorded. It should also be recorded in the parent-held child record and in a form which is then sent to the district community health computer input clerk.

From a practical point of view, this may cause difficulties because the child health record does not usually appear in the parent's hands until after the first visit by the health visitor. Therefore, it may be necessary to supply to the parents an additional page which can be inserted later into the child health record in the appropriate place or copied into the record by the health visitor at the time of his/her assessment.

Computerisation of the record

The only purpose of the district computer is that it can marry up every registered birth with every clinical examination and this means that, in theory, there could be a very simple way of determining whether or not every baby has been screened for DDH. Unless every baby is screened, the system is bound to fail. Computer software is such that it would be very easy to be alerted if any birth appeared on the computer without there being the appropriate screening examination entered within the first 2 weeks of life.

The great importance of this will be emphasised at the time of secondary screening. This occurs at the age of 6–8 weeks and is not always done by the same individual. It is likely to be the GP or the clinical medical officer but the method of examination and recording should be the same and that information should be fed back into the computerised record held at the district level. The same alarm system could be used to detect any child that has not undergone this secondary screening procedure.

Needless to say, if ultrasound is part of the system in any particular area, then of course this also can be fed back into the system.

Ultimately, a computer record will give meaningful information that will confirm that 100% of the birth population has been screened, and not only that they have been screened but that they have been screened at the right times. The computer record input is such that all the appropriate questions must be asked and all the appropriate observations on examination must be done, for an entry is required on each square of the questionnaire.

The importance of the designated officer is in the feedback which completes the audit loop (Figure 9.2). The computerised information should be reviewed regularly by the designated officer so that he/she is immediately aware of cases which are not being screened and is also immediately aware of cases which present to an orthopaedic department with a late stage of the disease. The officer is then in a position to check this out against the record of screening so that information can be fed back to the primary screeners.

This of course is the main argument against the primary screeners being a population of professionals who change at regular intervals. It is much better for these primary screeners to be relatively permanent posts and this is one of the main reasons why, say, a paediatric physiotherapist is more suitable than a paediatric junior doctor.

Audit

This subject was discussed by Jones *et al.* in 1991. It is most important that the audit loop is completed as shown in Figure 9.2. There must be feedback in order that the learning process occurs, and it is said to be the function of the designated officer to provide this feedback.

At present, however, there is little purpose in feedback as a method of education because the nature of the work of senior house officers is that

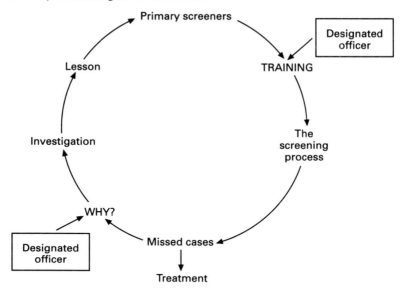

Figure 9.2 The audit loop being completed for screening. It will be noted that the designated officer has a function in training and asking 'why?' if cases are overlooked. The officer also has a function in the overall administration of the process and has to check that all the susceptible population are actually examined. (See Figure 9.2.)

by the time the information has been fed back they have usually progressed in their training process to a different job. Nevertheless, the doctor or the screener should be informed, in order that they can benefit from the learning experience. Unfortunately the system is not going to benefit if the screeners regularly change their jobs.

There is a strong case for a formal audit meeting with the administrators of the audit process together with the screeners on a regular monthly or bimonthly basis in each health district. It is important that the records are computerised in such a way that an automatic check is made, firstly, on whether all the population are being screened and, secondly, whether the whole population is returning for subsequent screening examinations. This is outlined in the algorithm in Figure 9.3.

A typical monthly audit report might be expected to record the information in Figure 9.4.

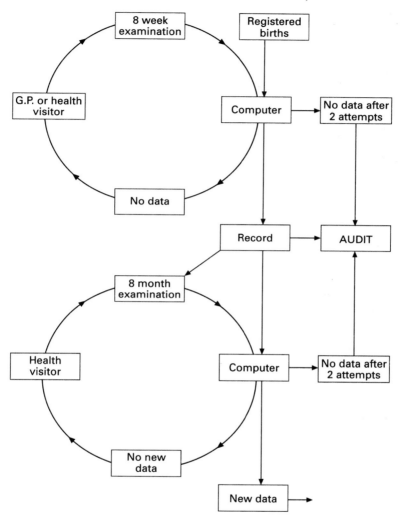

Figure 9.3 Algorithm demonstrating how audit can work at each screening period. The first cycle is the 8-week examination and the second cycle the 9-month examination. The computer needs to check that all registered births receive an examination and if they have not that should be instituted. Where a successful record comes out of this process that record should then be fed into the 8-month examination cycle and again a computer check should be made to make sure that the appropriate data is recorded. It is important that the administration of the system checks that all babies are examined at 8 weeks and that all babies are examined at 8 months.

1.	Number of births	=	A
2.	Number of babies examined	=	B
3.	If B<A		Review missing records next month
4.	Number of positives		
5.	Number splinted		
6.	Number of babies in the 'high risk' group	=	C
7.	Number of babies scanned	=	D
8.	If C>D		Investigate unscanned cases
9.	Number of babies requiring intervention (e.g. plaster cast or surgery) during same period		

Figure 9.4 A typical monthly audit report.

References

Jones, D.A., Beynon, D. and Littlepage, B.N. (1991). Audit of an official recommendation on screening for congenital dislocation of the hip. *Br. Med. J.*, **302**, 1435–1436.

Further reading

Davies, S.J. and Walker, G. (1984). Problems in the early recognition of hip dysplasia. *J. Bone Joint Surg.*, **66B**, 479–484.

Klisic, P., Zivanovic, V. and Brdar, R. (1988). Effects of triple prevention of CDH, stimulated by distribution of 'baby packages'. *J. Paediat. Orthop.*, **8**, 9–11.

Salter, R. (1968). Etiology, pathogenesis and possible prevention of congenital dislocation of the hip. *Can. Med. Assoc. J.*, **98**, 933–945.

SUGGESTED FURTHER READING

General

Jones, D.A. (1994). Principles of screening and congenital dislocation of the hip. *Ann. R. Coll. Surg. Engl.*, **76**, 245–250.

McKeown, T. and Lowe, C.R. (1966). *An Introduction to Social Medicine.* Oxford: Blackwell.

Palmen, K. (1984). Prevention of congenital dislocation of the hip. The Swedish experience of neonatal treatment of hip joint instability. *Acta Orthop. Scand. Suppl.*, **208**, 1–107.

Standing Medical Advisory Committee, Standing Nursing and Midwifery Advisory Committee for the Secretaries of State for Social Services and for Wales (1986). *Screening for the Detection of Congenital Dislocation of the Hip.* London: Department of Health and Social Security.

Tonis, D. (1987). *Congenital Dysplasia and Dislocation of the Hip in Children and Adults.* Berlin: Springer Verlag.

Wilkinson, J.A. (1985). *Congenital Displacement of the Hip Joint.* Berlin: Springer Verlag.

Wilson, J. and Junger, G. (1968). *Principles and Practice of Screening for Disease.* Geneva: World Health Organisation.

Index